THE NEUROSURGICAL APPROACH
TO INTRACRANIAL INFECTIONS

A REVIEW OF PERSONAL EXPERIENCES 1940 - 1960

BY

F. J. IRSIGLER, M.D.

FOREWORD BY

PROFESSOR H. OLIVECRONA
STOCKHOLM

WITH 67 FIGURES

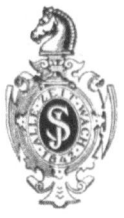

Springer-Verlag Berlin Heidelberg GmbH

1961

ISBN 978-3-662-22987-3   ISBN 978-3-662-24936-9 (eBook)
DOI 10.1007/978-3-662-24936-9

DEDICATED TO

GERNOT BRUNO IRSIGLER

A STUDENT OF THE MEDICAL SCHOOL
AT THE WITWATERSRAND UNIVERSITY

Foreword

The introduction of antibiotics has practically eliminated infection of the paranasal sinuses as source of intracranial infections. Thoracic surgery has nearly eradicated a formerly fairly frequent source of abscess of the brain, namely infections of the lung, such as lung abscess, bronchiectasia and lung gangrene. Gunshot wounds of the head are of course a very important course of brain abscess and meningitis, but in civilian practice fortunately rare. Complicated fractures of the vault and fractures of the base of the skull are at present the most important source of intracranial infection, and are likely to increase in importance due to ever increasing frequency of motor accidents. Metastatic brain abscess originating from a focus of infection of the tonsils or from other lesions anywhere in the body are on the whole rare. This source of infection must be considered to be of minor importance.

These facts are clearly reflected in Dr. IRSIGLER's monograph. There is an abundance of material of traumatic abscesses both due to gunshot wounds and to peace-time accidents involving the vault, the base of the skull and the paranasal sinuses, which is extensively documented by case histories and well chosen illustrations.

One should have liked some information on electro-encephalograms in cases of brain abscess in the acute and chronic stage, but absence of comments on this particular aspect of the subject is probably due to the fact that a good deal of the material was collected before electroencephalograms were routinely made and before the importance of this type of examination was fully realized. Echoencephalograms were not yet invented when the author collected his material, but it is to be hoped that this type of examination will be used in a future revision of his book.

I have enjoyed reading Dr. IRSIGLER's book and it is to be recommended to every neurosurgeon, especially because of its wealth of valuable information concerning the relation between head injury and intracranial infection.

Stockholm, September 2, 1960

Acknowledgements

My sincerest thanks go to Professor W. Tönnis, former Director of the Neurosurgical University Clinic at the Charité in Berlin, and to Professor H. Krayenbühl, Director of the Neurosurgical University Clinic in Zürich. At these two clinics I trained and worked during the first half of the period covered by the present monograph. The majority of cases included here I witnessed and operated on at these clinics. In other cases, mainly those in Zürich, I had the privilege of assisting at their operations. Most of the clinical and pathological data are from my own records.

In 1951, when I came to South Africa, Mr. R. A. Kraynauw, F.R.C.S.,formerly leading neurosurgeon in Johannesburg, provided me with ample opportunity to keep in touch with the neurosurgical field during the ensuing years.

During my work at the General Hospital in Pretoria (1955—1957) I saw and operated on many cases of all kinds of cranio-cerebral trauma and its sequelae, and on pyogenic and fungal infections of the central nervous system which are so common among the native population of this country. The experiences gained are incorporated in the present monograph to form a supplement and counterpart to those encountered on the Continent and during the last war.

Finally, a number of cases are presented here which, together with Mr. M. J. Joubert, F.R.C.S., I had the opportunity to see and operate on during recent years at various hospitals in Durban and Pietermaritzburg, Natal. Thanks are due to him and to the medical superintendents of these hospitals.

I have been both honoured and encouraged by Professor Olivecrona's willingness to write a foreword to this volume.

All photographs come from the skilful hands of Mr. Theo Marais, head of the photographic department, Pretoria University.

My own rough sketches which underlie the figures 7, 22, 58, 60, 64, and 66, have been transformed into brilliant drawings by the graphic art of Mr. H. P. Weber from the Neurosurgical University Clinic in Zürich.

Mr. A. N. Boyce, M. A., Krugersdorp, was kind enough to read the manuscript and give most valuable advice on the English phraseology.

My wife assisted me in compiling the subject index and the bibliography; more than this: she was my most devoted companion during our pilgrimage from war-stricken Berlin to this town on the West Rand, which bears the name of a great figure in South African history.

The publishers, Springer-Verlag, have done their best to maintain the high standard of their world-wide reputation.

Krugersdorp in the Transvaal — June, 1960   F. J. Irsigler

Contents

Introduction

Points in differential diagnosis

In this introductory survey some of the more uncommon features will be considered which may give, and in fact have given, rise, in the present series, to differential diagnostic considerations such as to the presence at all, and the possible type of a pyogenic intracranial condition.

1. Thrombosis and thrombophlebitis of dural sinuses and cerebral veins

The presence of a tangle of thrombosed veins related to a brain abscess which has been excised in toto, may give some hint as to the etiology and pathogenesis of such an abscess; the same is true with dural sinus thrombosis following fronto-basal injury or associated with rhinogenous subdural empyema; they all will be considered in Chapter A (cases 1.1, 1.2, 1.7, 1.17). However, such instances may seem isolated and singular, and hardly bear out the general correlation between pyogenic intracranial lesions of surgical proportions and affection of intracranial venous channels with which we are now concerned.

If we accept SYMONDS (1952) dictum that "intracranial venous thrombosis may be complicating any infective focus however trivial and wherever situated in the body", it should be realised that the same is true for any kind of intracranial infection including subdural empyema and brain abscess. It is then obvious that differential diagnostic considerations here gain practical importance within the field of the neurosurgeon.

For clinical convenience it is feasible to adopt PENNYBACKER's (1945) classification of intracranial venous thrombosis into the following two conditions:

1. Obstruction, more commonly of transient type, of the larger dural channels such as the superior longitudinal and the lateral sinuses, with rapidly increasing intracranial pressure resulting, if not relieved adequately and in time, in ventricular dilatation. Obstruction of the arachnoid villi (SYMONDS, 1937) and tributaries draining into the sinuses may well be a contributory factor in some cases. As a rule, there are no localising features and advanced papilloedema may be in contrast with a good general appearance of the patient. The most prominent condition here is the so-called otitic hydrocephalus (SYMONDS, 1931) which will be discussed more fully in Chapter C in connection with the otogenous class.

I have seen three cases of *superior sagittal sinus thrombosis* during recent years. All three followed injury to the head. In two patients there was a scalp wound and depressed fracture overlying that sinus; in one patient the wound healed per primary union whereas it turned septic in the other case resulting in a localised subdural and, probably, interhemispherical abscess which, nevertheless, was drained successfully. In the third patient who had sustained a blow with a stick to his right fronto-parietal area without bony involvement, a left hemiplegia developed quite suddenly four months after the injury, and remained stationary after that. A right carotid angiogram revealed, in the late venous phase, obstruction of the superior sagittal sinus involving its anterior part as far back as the rolandic region. The pictures were interpreted as indicating a mural thrombosis.

All three patients had a left hemiplegia with considerable spasticity and involving, in one, the proximal parts of the limbs more than the distal parts; in one patient there was paraplegia of both legs from which he recovered slowly. As is well known from missile wounds involving the mid-sagittal region and not infrequently seen during the last war, the bladder may be or may not be affected; if it is, the term *"Mantelkantensyndrom"* has been applied to the clinical picture by German authors[1]. This, if associated with paraplegia of the legs, is very likely to be misinterpreted as spinal cord injury. Only in one of the three patients under discussion, a Bantu woman of about thirty, a lasting bladder incontinence was observed right from the beginning, and requiring an indwelling catheter. In none of the patients convulsions of any sort were recorded.

2. The second type of intracranial venous involvement comprises localised venous thrombosis or thrombophlebitis of cortical or smaller dural sinus tributaries with clinical evidence of local cortical irritation such as jacksonian or adversive attacks, occasionally revealing a definite "march of discharge" as described by MITCHELL (1952) in children. In cases where the venous channels on the base of the brain are affected certain types of cranial nerve palsies are diagnostic and due to pressure from the clot to the adjacent nerves. The classical example here is the cavernous sinus syndrome of which an example will be given later (case 1.21 in Chapter A). Most conspicuous, however, and of equal practical import is unilateral or bilateral 6th nerve paresis described by SYMONDS (1952), WEBER (1957) and others. GRADENIGO's syndrome, viz. one-sided paresis of the external rectus oculi associated with either acute or chronic middle ear infection, belongs to the group under consideration and has been interpreted, since GRADENIGO's original description in 1907, in various ways from the point of morbid anatomy. Since rapid and complete recovery frequently occurs, apparently due to recanalisation or venous by-pass, a localised venous thrombosis is likely to be the underlying cause as suggested by SYMONDS in 1952. In at least a number of cases classified as GRADENIGO's syndrome the channels involved most probably are the system of inferior petrosal sinuses adjacent to DORELLO's canal, and draining into the internal jugular vein, or, more specifically, as advanced by COURVILLE (1950), the veins draining the tip of the petrous bone.

In the absence of signs of present, as well as history of past, ear infection the etiology of isolated 6th nerve palsy often remains obscure especially if signs of raised intracranial pressure or additional intracranial pathology are lacking. This was the case in an Indian woman of 29 who had developed, two months prior to examination, a right-sided parietal headache extending into the right supraocular and ocular regions, occasional vomiting and watering of the right eye and right nostril. Somewhat later, she started complaining of increasingly annoying diplopia which was found due to paresis of the right external rectus muscle. There was no agreement, among the examiners, as to the presence of facial weakness and involvement of the third nerve; the right upper lid seemed to droop. All other findings including the lumbar fluid and complement reaction for syphilis were negative. The skull including the base had been carefully examined radiologically and bilateral carotid angiograms had been done, no pathology was found. The otologist was unable to find anything wrong in her ears and acoustic nerves. Since the patient had undergone already extensive X-ray studies when seen first, an air encephalogram was postponed; however, she failed to turn up for re-assessment.

In quite a number of GRADENIGO's 57 cases, there were, in addition to abducens nerve palsy, also signs of involvement of the anterior group of cranial nerves such as the trigeminal, oculomotor and even the optic nerves. SYMONDS (1952) has mentioned a rare involvement of the motor division of the trigeminal nerve consequent to superior petrosal sinus thrombosis. On the whole, however, involvement of the trigeminal nerve means either extension into the cavernous sinus or, especially in cases with insidious onset and slow progression of symptoms, neoplastic infiltration of the base of skull. We shall return to this in Section 2. It should be emphasized here that some confusion has arisen in using the term "GRADENIGO's syndrome" because, since GRADENIGO's original paper in 1907,

---

[1] In World War I, a "longitudinal sinus syndrome" has been described by HOLMES and SARGENT in Brit. Med. J. 2, 493 (1915).

various signs related to cranial nerves have been added later; it had become clear also that the pathology underlying this condition is by no means a single and well-defined one. Consequently, GRADENIGO's syndrome now cannot be regarded as a morbid entity of its own. The clinical picture and the pathology of suppuration of the petrous pyramid, more specifically of its tip, has been elaborated comprehensively in a series of papers by KO-PETZKY and ALMOUR in 1930—1931.

3. To the foregoing two types of intracranial venous thrombosis a third one should be added where cerebral thrombophlebitis, often preceded by some kind of constitutional infection presents as a morbid entity of its own and of sufficient severity. A detailed clinical description of this type has been given by KRAYENBÜHL and WEBER (1952) and WEBER (1957). Although I myself have not come across this condition it is set out here for differential-diagnostic reasons.

In striking contrast to the two types just described the patients with cortical thrombophlebitis give at once the clinical impression of being acutely and severely ill. The condition often masquerades acute brain abscess the differential diagnosis from which may be both difficult and decisive regarding the patient's survival. As a rule, the lesion responds well to chemotherapy and expectant treatment whereas anticoagulants (suggested by KRAYENBÜHL and WEBER) would seem of doubtful value in view of the tendency to intracerebral bleeds associated, on attempts to operative removal, with increasing pressure indicative of malignant cerebral oedema. This sequence of events is well demonstrated by one of the cases from the Zürich Clinic. Lastly, the condition may conceal *a quiescent* brain abscess which unexpectedly may rupture into the ventricle. Explorative needling and ventriculography are ill-advised and, instead, repeated angiograms are indicated. Since detailed histology is as yet lacking it remains debatable whether the condition is related to or even identical with the sort of suppurative encephalitis decribed by BOTTERELL and DRAKE (1952). KRAYENBÜHL and WEBER, in one of their cases, excised a piece, 2 cm. long, of an obstructed cortical vein[1].

There is yet another reason for advising against ventriculography in suspected cortical thrombophlebitis: the air pictures may be misleading. It has been pointed out by PENNY-BACKER (1945) and confirmed by KRAYENBÜHL and WEBER (1952) that purulent cerebral thrombophlebitis may cause a definite shift of the ventricular system to the opposite side thus suggesting, falsely, presence of a cerebral abscess.

On the whole, it is true, an increased bulk of one cerebral hemisphere with consequent displacement beneath the falx cerebri will rightly favour the diagnosis of cerebral abscess; however, the shift may be entirely out of proportion regarding size of the abscess (or small abscesses). This was the case in a woman of 51, who, two months following a bilateral frontal leucotomy through button hole trephine openings, developed a sudden hemiplegia on the left. The air encephalogram disclosed a pronounced shift of the lateral ventricles and the 3rd ventricle to the left side, and flattening of the roof of the right lateral ventricle. There was air in the basal cistern, within the right temporal horn as well as in the right sylvian fossa and all three were displaced to the left. There was no papilloedema, and the lumbar fluid was clear and under normal pressure. There was significant puffy oedema of the scalp in front of the incision on right. Re-exploration on the right side revealed the dura mater under high tension and the brain protruding like toothpaste through the hole in the dura. Needling with the brain cannula in various directions yielded only a few drops of thick pus from a soft, spongy brain. On the left, the dura mater was under normal tension. The patient recovered slowly and was reported, 6 weeks afterwards, as walking

---

[1] The reader is referred to the papers by R. GARCIN et M. PESTEL, Thrombo-phlébites cérébrales. Paris: Masson et Cie. 1949, and H. KRAYENBÜHL, Cerebral venous Thrombosis, in Schweiz. Arch. f. Neurol. u. Psychiat. 74, 261 (1955). The value of electro-encephalography in diagnosis of cerebral thrombophlebitis has been stressed by L. CHRISTOPHE, Thrombophlébites cérébrales et neurochirurgie, in Presse méd. 59, 1194 (1951), and by T. HAHN, Die Elektroencephalographie bei cerebralen Thrombophlebitiden und Thrombosen. Inaug-Diss. Zürich 1954.

with two sticks, talking sensibly and with appropriate facial expression; there was a fair control of bladder and bowels.

It is generally held that in cases like this the increased bulk of the hemisphere involved is due to cerebral oedema surrounding comparatively small deposits of pus; however, the part played by concomitant cerebral thrombophlebitis is not yet clear.

2. Tumours of the base of skull

In the present context tumours involving the base of skull will be mentioned only briefly. They gain neurosurgical interest at three sites: the paranasal sinuses, the middle fossa, more specifically the parasellar region, and finally the petrous bone. Chapter A will be devoted to rhinogenous pathology. Parasellar tumours will be discussed in Section 3 together with vascular anomalies within the cavernous sinus. Thus, we are left with the petrous bone. Tumours arising at this site enter the neurosurgical field in a way which will be illustrated in the following case history. The differential diagnosis from sequelae of chronic ear infection and thrombosis of the adjacent veins may be somewhat precarious and usually requires cooperation with the aural surgeon.

Case 0.1. Neuroblastoma of the petrous bone in a 4-year-old child presenting with a Gradenigo-like syndrome which progressed rapidly to involve the bulk of the cranial nerves on the side of the affected ear. Mistakenly, a mastoidectomy was carried out. Intracranial suppuration was ruled out by air studies. Punch biopsy from a "polyp" growing within the external auditory meatus. No operation. Death followed temporary improvement, 4 months after onset of illness.

This was a female child of 4 who started complaining of left-sided ear ache, about six weeks prior to admission; shortly afterwards a squint and a weakness of the left half of her face was noticed. There was no discharge from the ear. Nearly three weeks after the onset of symptoms, a left mastoidectomy was carried out. The findings were essentially negative. The dura mater was exposed and some granulations were scraped off. No histology was done. The dural surgeon in performing this operation admittedly felt "not at all happy" about what he had found. A gauze wick was inserted for drainage but again, there was no discharge from the ear; X-rays were reported to disclose erosion of the tip of the left petrous bone and some query calcarious deposits above it.

On admission to the ward the child was listless and utterly non-coöperative. She was running a temperature but her neck was supple. The left mastoid region was tender and seemed slightly bulging. The mastoid incision was in process of healing and there was slight brownish discharge on the gauze wick. We managed to visualise the left fundus which showed no papilloedema. There was complete peripheral facial paralysis on the left and an internal squint of the left eye. The pupils were about equal and there was no obvious nystagmus. There seemed to be a hypoaesthesia of the left half of her face and her tongue slightly deviated to the left. She was to all probability deaf in her left ear.

We were not sure about a weakness of her left arm and leg but slight incoördination of the left arm was present. Repeated X-rays (Fig. 1) confirmed the previous findings of an erosion of the left petrous bone in so far as the upper margin of the tip showed interruption of its contour and there was also lessened density of the bone structure. No calcifications could be detected in relation to this area. This picture is clearly different from that found in suppuration of the petrous apex as elaborated by TAYLOR (1931) whose description is derived from RÖNTGEN findings in patients under the care of KOPETZKY and ALMOUR; their papers have been referred to earlier (p. 3). The lumbar fluid was normal in every respect. An air encephalogram was done and revealed a nice filling of all ventricles and the subarachnoid spaces, avobe and below the tentorium. There was no shift and the left temporal horn was normal with regard to its shape and position; so was the fourth ventricle. The great cistern was also filled with air.

At this stage we were left with the tentative diagnosis of petrositis of the left temporal bone especially its apical portion, associated with a neurological syndrome indicating, in keeping with GRADENIGO's description, ipsilateral abducens and trigeminal involvement which, however, in the course of some weeks, already had extended to involve additionally the caudal group of the cranial nerves including the facial and hypoglossus; even some signs of ipsilateral cerebellar involvement were present. There was no discharge from the ear and no pleocytosis in the lumbar fluid. All signs were confined to the left side. A brain abscess, either above or below the tentorium, was ruled out by air studies.

On giving intravenous terramycin the temperature returned to normal within a few days; neurologically, there was no change. During the third week of her hospital stay, however, definite signs of progression became apparent: there was now a complete left ophthalmoplegia with the left pupil maximally dilated and fixed, and a suggestion of protrusion of the left eye. It was impossible to establish beyond doubt sensory loss in the left half of her face in this resistent child. Additionally, her voice had become husky and her speech dysarthric. Signs of dysphagia developed, too. There was query wasting of the left half of her tongue. Finally, there was gross atrophy of the left sternocleidomastoid muscle. The neck glands on the left were enlarged so as to be palpable, and hard. Under general anaesthesia, the physical examination could be completed and, first of all, a pale, soft, non-haemorrhagic "polyp" was diclosed obstructing the left auditory meatus. A punch biopsy was done by Dr. R. Gowans. The nasopharynx, on inspection, revealed no tumor. Tissue was taken from the left nasopharynx and, under the microscope, proved to be of normal lymphatic structure. The vocal cords could not be visualised clearly; but there could be little doubt as to paralysis of the left recurrent nerve. Finally, fundoscopy revealed a normal fundus on the right, whereas on the left, there was some haziness and the cup appeared filled.

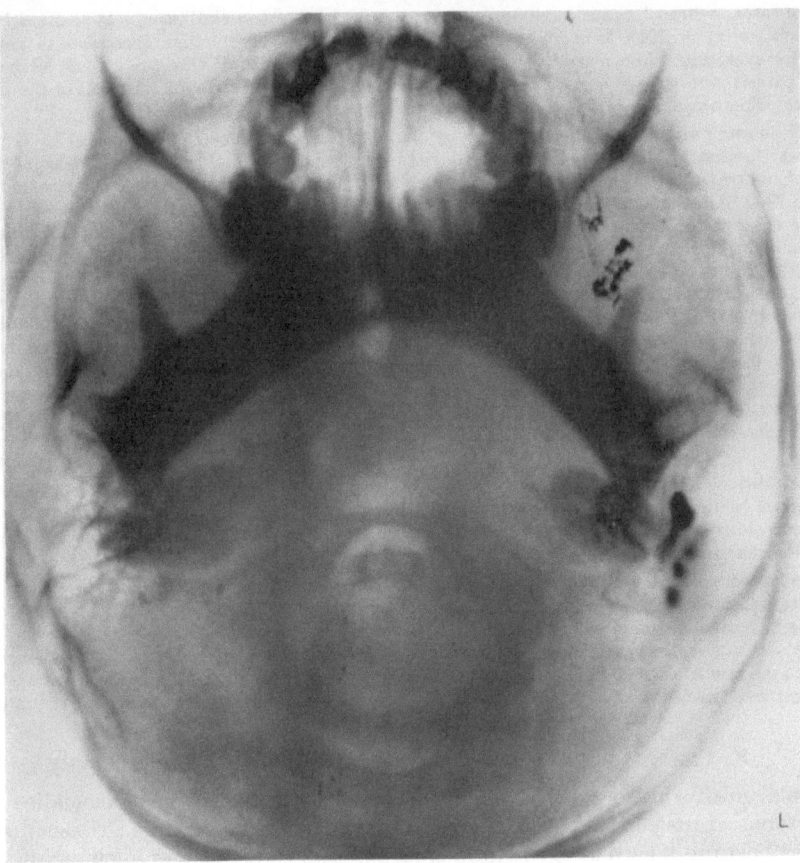

Fig. 1. Radiological appearance of the base of skull to show the petrous bones in a child, aged 4, with a neuro-blastoma of the left pyramid. Diagnosis was made from biopsy from a polyp within the left aural meatus. Osteitis of the petrous bone was first suspected and intracranial abscess ruled out by air encephalography. (Case O.1). Note iodoform deposits in left mastoid region

Histologically, the tumour from the left auditory meatus appeareed to be a relatively anaplastic neuro-blastoma with round and spindle-shaped cells and fairly numerous mitoses. There was a dense reticulum pattern and perivascular palisading was apparent.

The child improved considerably under vitamin B_{12} and deep therapy, and was subsequently taken to Rhodesia where she died, approximately 4 months after the onset of her illness. It was reported that she was full of secondaries and had much pain in the last. It is unknown whether some adrenal tumour has been ascertained.

Comment. Here, the familiar picture of unilateral ear ache and sixth nerve paresis was soon complicated by a peripheral facial paralysis which apparently indicated that we were dealing with something more serious than a localised apical petrous suppuration supposed to underlie, in some of the cases at least, a gradenigo-like picture. The temperature after her admission to the hospital made the differential diagnosis by no means easier. The main issue, of course, was to rule out an intracranial suppuration related to the affected ear. This question was conclusively answererd in the negative by the normal air encephalogram. However, the neoplastic nature of the lesion became apparent only when, together with the mass in the left aural meatus, the neck glands on the side of the involved ear were found hardened and enlarged. By this time, it is true, the tumour had already grown so far as to involve the third cranial nerve but still remained confined to the one side.

The presenting syndrome bore some similarity to the so-called TROTTER's *triad or sinus of Morgagni syndrome* as seen in tumours of the lateral nasopharyngeal wall; it is characterised by deafness, trigeminal involvement and paralysis of the palate; later the neck glands become enlarged; not infrequently, a 6th nerve paralysis is seen too (ASHERSON, ORMEROD). In our case the nasopharynx was thoroughly examined and a biopsy done from that site; normal lymphatic tissue was found.

In rare cases, a branchiogenic carcinoma may reach the base of the skull as in a 14-year-old boy reported on by CORREA et al. in 1947. As in our case, ear ache, fever and the radiological appearance of petrositis were present. However, apart from a nasal voice the cranial nerves were intact. One surely would have expected an abducens paresis, the more so because necrotic material had been removed from the point of the petrous bone during mastoidectomy.

Finally, in our patient, an aberrant *tumour of the carotid body* or, to use the term coined by GUILD (quoted from ROSENWASSER, vide infra), a glomus jugulare tumour had to be considered a remote possibility. The first instance of an erratic carotid body tumour involving the middle ear and petrous bone was reported by ROSENWASSER in 1945. Another example was published by C. M. PROWSE in 1958, just at the time when our patient was under observation. PROWSE's case, a 47-year-old European woman, had complained of lancinating ear ache on the right side and several attempts had been made to remove a polyp from the right middle ear, every attempt being followed by profuse haemorrhage; all cranial nerves on the right from the 5th to the 12th, both included, were palsied; the long tracts were involved too, at first on the left, later also on the right side. X-rays showed a moth-eaten destruction of the right petrous bone, including its tip, and extending into the right jugular foramen and towards the condylar fossa, with islands of intact bone preserved; the picture suggested an extremely vascular lesion in keeping with the clinical appearance. The patient improved markedly on deep X-ray therapy. — The case shows that glomus jugulare tumours, because of their close anatomical relationship to the petrous temporal bone, are likely to disclose their neoplastic nature early in history. Consequently the question of intracranial pyogenic complication will seldom arise [1].

KESSLER et al., in 1957, reported on a rare case of *cavernoma* of the petrous pyramid in a child of 8 who had clinical and radiological signs of mastoiditis and was admitted with a diagnosis of brain abscess. The roentgenogram included in the paper, shows significant patchy sclerosing of the right petrous bone which is in striking contrast to the bone destruction in both neuroblastoma and glomus jugulare tumour. The child died from epidural haemorrhage.

In order to complete this discussion on tumours of the cranium, it may be mentioned here, that the present writer twice was faced with secondaries from adrenal neuroblastoma in patients under investigation for brain abscess. In the case discussed above, the base of the skull was involved. The other instance was an infant presenting with a localised swelling on the forehead which gave the impression of a subaponeurotic abscess exactly like the one in case 1.6 from which a frontal abscess was removed (p. 20). In the infant mentioned, all clinical signs were in favour of a neuroblastoma, but post mortem confirmation could not be obtained.

3. Cavernous sinus syndrome in subclinoid carotid anomaly

Vascular malformations such as berry aneurysms or arterio-venous anomalies involving the cavernous sinus portion of the carotid artery commonly produce a classical syndrome which has become known as cavernous sinus syndrome and allows to pin-point the lesion rather safely. JEFFERSON, in his paper in 1938, even made an attempt to sub-classify the syndrome corresponding to the more anterior or posterior site of the lesion within the cavernous sinus. In practice, there is considerable overlap and from the point of view of surgical approach it does not make much difference whether the lesion is placed more anteriorly or posteriorly so that such refinement in diagnosis is mainly of theoretical interest. JEFFERSON, himself, did not attempt to correlate the neurological symptoms with any definite kind of intracranial approach in the two cases out of 17 where such approach has been deemed feasible. What is of more concern here is the differential diagnosis from cavernous sinus thrombosis required in cases of acute onset and rapid progression of unilateral or bilateral neurological signs; in the absence of a murmur, pulsating exophthalmos, and bone destruction around the sella turcica and on the base of the cranium, the neurological diagnosis becomes both difficult and imperative. Twining's erosion of the superior i.e. sphenoidal orbital fissure and the wall of the optic foramen if carefully sought for, as first shown by JEFFERSON (1938), may well give conclusive evi-

---

[1] A comprehensive study on carotid body tumours is presented by O. KLEINSASSER in: Handbuch der Neurochirurgie, herausgeg. von H. OLIVECRONA u. W. TÖNNIS, Bd. IV, Erster Teil, Pathologie des Geschwülste des Hirnschädels, p. 466 et seq. Berlin: Springer 1960.

dence of an aneurysm. The diagnostic procedure par excellence, however, is carotid angiography. As to the differential diagnosis from brain abscess Jefferson in his paper remarks that cavernous aneurysms previously have been misdiagnosed and operated on as abscesses. "Such experiences may yet befall others".

The following case history will serve to exemplify various points in diagnosis and differential diagnosis of the lesions.

Case 0.2. Rapidly progressing cavernous sinus syndrome in a woman of 47 with what was interpreted, on the carotid angiogram, as a non-fistulous intracavernous vascular anomaly. Death followed placing of a silver clip on and muscle-plugging of, the aneurysm in loco.

This was an Indian woman of 47 with a short story of left-sided hemicrania resulting, within a few days, in her inability to open at first her left, soon afterwards also her right eye. The pain became localised at the top and in the middle of the head, and was of increasing severity.

Neurologically, there was bilateral complete ophthalmoplegia and ptosis but no chemosis of the conjunctivae. The fundi were normal and there was no visual defect. There was a query bilateral exophthalmos without any signs of pulsation. There was, in addition, loss of sensation in the 1st division of the left trigeminal nerve. No clinical signs of pituitary involvement were present and the rest of the neurological examination was within normal.

X-rays of the skull revealed a normal sella turcica with minute calcareous deposits behind the dorsum sellae and possibly projecting into the pituitary fossa itself. There was no apparent destruction on the base of the cranium nor any erosion around the sphenoidal fissure.

A carotid angiogram was first carried out on the left i.e. the side of trigeminal involvement. A non-fistulous vascular anomaly was disclosed occupying the infraclinoid portion of the carotid artery (Fig. 2). There was

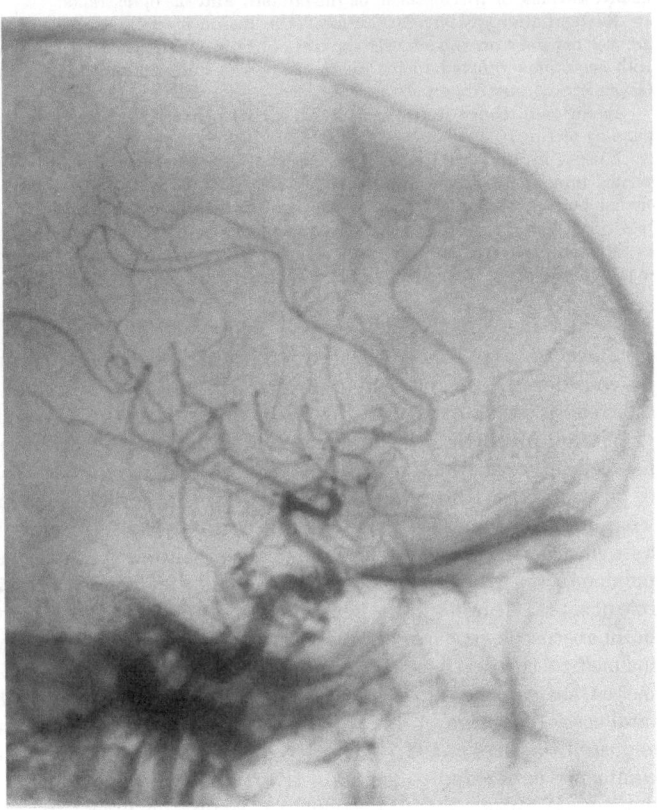

Fig. 2. Left carotid angiogram (lateral view), in a woman, aged 47, with a bilateral ophthalmoplegia and involvement of the 1st trigeminal division on the left. The picture was interpreted as an arterio-venous anomaly within but not communicating with, the cavernous sinus. (Case 0.2)

some argument as to its nature whether this was a saccular aneurysm or rather an arteriovenous malformation. It was argued that no venous channels draining the lesion were demonstrated on the phlebogram. A solid tumour within the cavernous sinus such as previously described by Dandy (1937) and Jefferson (1938) was considered as an alternative possibility. The anterior and sylvian groups were filled well but appeared somewhat thinned out. There was, however, overflow across the midline so much as to visualize clearly the right anterior cerebral. A right carotid angiogram revealed that the anomaly on the left was not fed from the right carotid system; again no draining channels could be discerned. *On exposure* through a left fronto-temporal osteoplastic flap the dura mater was found rather tense and so was the brain. There were no signs of recent or residua of previous subarachnoid bleed and a ventricular tap yielded clear fluid; upon this, the brain slacked down. The left optic nerve was found not displaced. Lateral to it and adjacent to the carotid artery there was an encapsulated, non-pulsatile, roundish mass of white-bluish colour occupying roughly the medial and anterior thirds of the middle fossa. Its estimated size was that of a pigeon's egg. The mass was covered by the dura mater which was continuous with that of the lesser sphenoidal wing in front of the mass. A long Olivecrona's aneurysmal silver clip was then placed on to the internal carotid (Dr. M. J. Joubert) alongside the optic nerve.

Tap with a thin needle yielded a few drops of arterial blood. On compression of the left carotid in the neck the intracranial aneurysm softened down slightly; while the compression was continued the capsule was incised and a gush of blood with some clots came up with considerable force but was soon brought under control with oxycel and and small grafts from the temporalis muscle. The dura was then closed tightly and the bone flap replaced. The patient, after receiving three pints of blood, came around while still on the table. The left eyeball now appeared somewhat softer as compared to the right and to the condition before the operation. A right hemiparesis was noticed. She died the following morning. No post mortem examination was granted.

Comment. The striking features in this case were: bilateral symmetrical involvement of the whole of external ocular muscles while the first trigeminal division was affected only on the left i.e. the side where the first neurological signs had appeared; the rapid progress so as to make surgery a matter of some urgency; finally, the lack of infringement on the chiasm and the optic tracts.

Bilateral angiography demonstrated the lesion precisely at the site where it was expected on neurological grounds but only on the left. The converse of this situation occurred in one of JEFFERSON's cases who presented with symptoms related to the cavernous sinus and confined to one side though suffering from a bilateral (asymmetrical) aneurysm at this site.

In our case, there were no signs of carotid-cavernous fistula and this possibly gives the clue to the puzzling picture.

DANDY, in 1937, described three cases of intracavernous lesion, two saccular aneurysms and one encapsulated tumour arising within the sinus; in all three patients he found the cavernous sinus obliterated precluding both development of an arterio-venous fistula and bleeding from the sinus. It seems likely that in the case cited above, an obliterative thrombosis of the cavernous sinus was present, too, and well to such extent as to cause pressure paralysis of the nerves traversing the sinus or its walls on either side without actual extension of the carotid anomaly to the opposite side.

4. Embolism

Since we are concerned here with intracranial infections mycotic embolism only will be considered, in relation to brain abscess and cerebral thrombosis. Emboli carrying infected material may reach the brain either from the heart or from any part of the systemic circulation including the pulmonary circulation. The importance of a patent foramen ovale has been overemphasized in the past and it is now widely held, mainly on the ground of post mortem findings, that patency of that foramen is not a condition sine qua non for what used to be called "paradoxical brain abscess". Apparently, clusters of microorganisms as well as crumbs of tissue up to a certain size may pass through the relatively wide pulmonary capillaries to lodge within the narrower capillaries of the brain. However, the role of septal defects in the heart is clearly demonstrated by the incidence of "paradoxical" brain abscesses in cases of congenital heart disease especially in FALLOT's tetralogy. One is inclined to think that a concomitant endocarditis may be the main source of bloodborne metastases. However, in none of the five patients with a brain abscess found among 115 fatal cases of congenital heart disease reported by GATES and coworkes in 1947 was there endocarditis present; it seems to follow that in congenital heart defects the infection commonly is carried to the brain from some silent focus within the systemic or pulmonary domain. WEBER, in 1957, collected from the literature 74 cases of brain abscess and cerebral venous thrombosis associated with congenital heart disease mainly FALLOT's tetratology. No case in point has been encountered in the present series.

The effects of embolism on the brain are not yet fully understood and probably more complex than previously was thought — even under the pure conditions of animal experiments. Certainly, not only structural changes occur as studied primarily so far. Arterial spasm, focal as well as generalized so as to involve distant areas of the brain, come into play resulting in secondary changes. Such reactive spasms reflect the intrinsic control of cerebral circulation and are reminiscent of (and possibly related to) the long-lasting arterial spasms following rupture of brain aneurysms where they can be visualized on angiograms and may well aggravate the clinical picture (NORLÉN and BARNUM, 1953).

In the case of mycotic embolism, additionally, some histolytic action of the microorganisms especially of the streptococcal group must be taken into account.

The effects of embolism in the brain can be classified roughly as follows:

1. Arterial obstruction. Several factors are involved in determining the site where an embolus comes to lodge. From experiments with air embolism (VILLARET and CACHERA,

1939) it is clear that the site of obstruction often is before or beyond a bifurcation. In septic embolism obstruction may or may not be followed by local destruction of the arterial wall (Fig. 3) with secondary haemorrhage into or abscess formation within the infarcted area. In order to rule out a suspected abscess exploration with the brain cannula or angiography may be called for, occasionally even more than once.

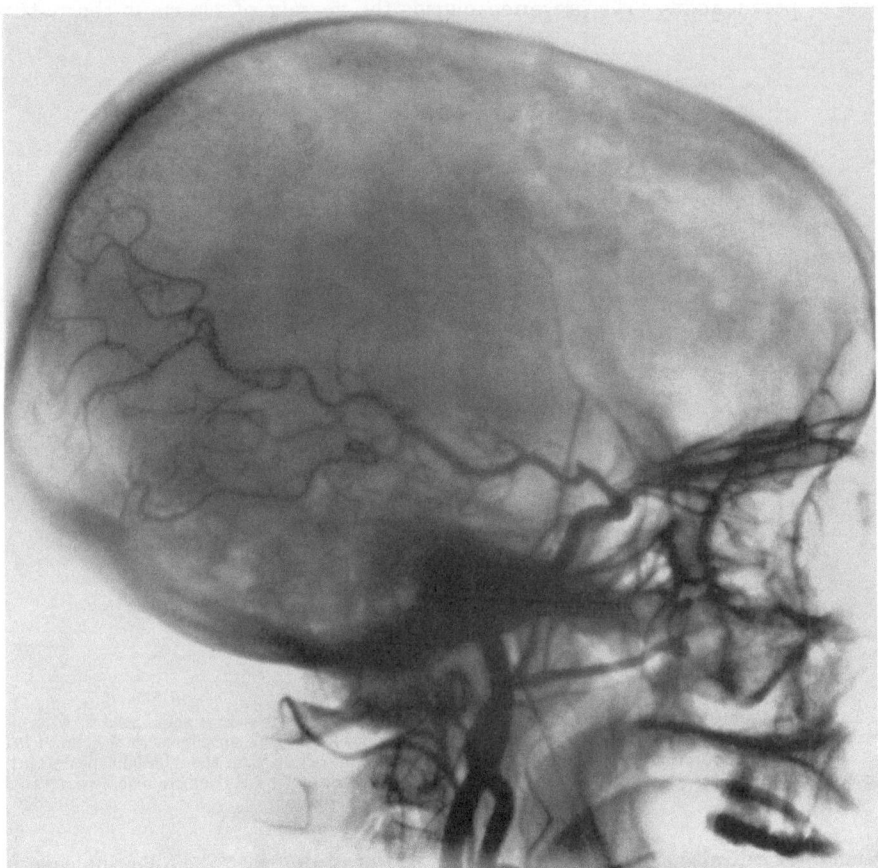

Fig. 3. Dentogenous embolic occlusion of the right sylvian artery just above the point of emergence of the posterior cerebral artery. Carotid angiogram 12 days after onset of symptoms which became apparent 3 days after extraction of a right lower molar tooth. There was no cardiac pathology. No abscess developed and the patient recovered but was left with a marked cerebral atrophy as evinced by air studies 7 weeks after onset

2. *Mycotic aneurysm* followed by haemorrhage, early or delayed, or by gross abscess formation. In subacute bacterial endocarditis both massive haemorrhage and gross abscess formation are uncommon occurrences; instead, a deep-seated infarction, on one or either side may be encountered on needling with the brain cannula in search for a suspected abscess (Fig. 4). Courville (1950) emphasized massive cerebral haemorrhage due to septic embolism from pelvic inflammation.

3. *Multiple septic embolisms* with miliary abscess formation following pyaemia such as from bacterial endocarditis (COURVILLE, 1950). This is a somewhat cumbrous terminology. A variety of lesions, microscopic in most cases, have been described such as endarteritis, foci of infarction and miliary abscesses around small vessels (DIAMOND). Whether the sequence of events resulting in such multiplicity of lesions is really initiated by the

avenue to the brain of infected emboli is a moot question. According to COURVILLE (1950) those emboli tend to lodge in the white matter of the brain whereas PETERS argues that they get stuck primarily within the brain cortex so much richer in capillaries than the white substance. Only exceptionally such emboli have been clearly demonstrated under the microscope e.g. by ISTOMANOVA[1] in 1928. What seems to be beyond doubt is changes in the wall of the small vessels, mainly the arterioles, followed, as one might surmise, by increase in permeability. The presence outside the vessels of plasma in the nature of a

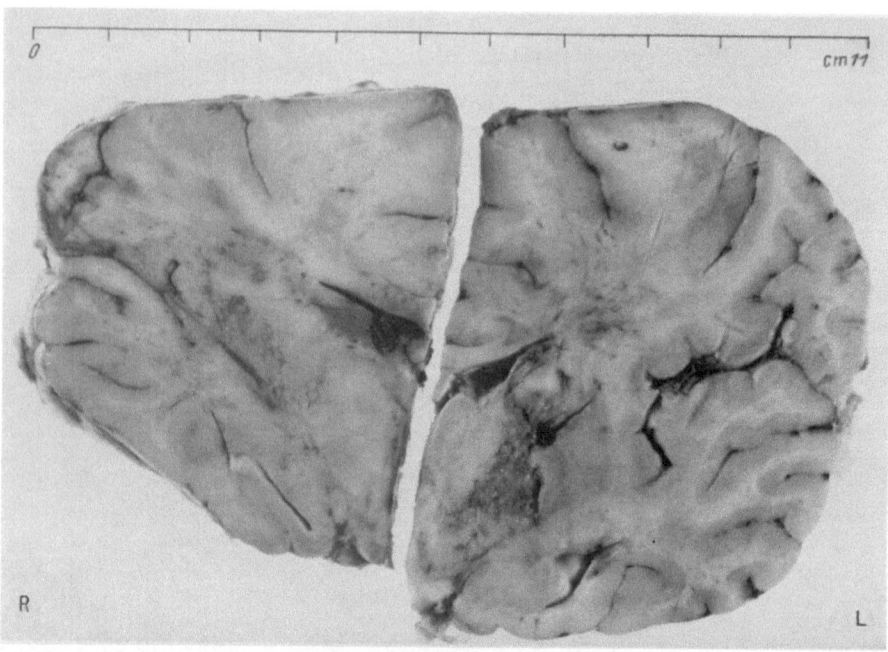

Fig. 4. Transverse sections through the right and left cerebral hemispheres in a child, aged 6, with subacute bacterial endocarditis. Streptococcus viridans was cultured from blood. The specimens show sylvian infarction of 2—3 weeks standing on right, and a recent haemorrhagic infarct occupying the internal capsule and part of basal ganglia on left. Exploration through burr holes was done on right to rule out brain abscess. (NB. The two sections are made in different planes)

transsudate or cellular exudate seems to be a matter of degree. The following case history is given in some detail to exemplify some of the points at issue as they are encountered not infrequently by the clinician.

Case 0.3. Signs of embolic involvement of the left cerebral hemisphere in a child of 12, with pyrexia, mitral incompetence most probably of rheumatic origin, and papilloedema. Ventricular catheter. No mycotic abscess found. Slow recovery.

An Indian girl of twelve was admitted to a district hospital in a semi-comatose state with the tentative diagnosis of typhoid fever and query meningitis. The lumbar fluid showed pleocytosis and at times there was a KERNIG's sign present. After a short-lived improvement she slipped into a state of restless confusion with high temperature. There was a pronounced bilateral papilloedema, a right-sided hemiparesis, aphasia and to all probability a hemianopic field defect to the right. The heart was grossly enlarged and there was a thrill and a hard systolic murmur over the apex — the impression was that of a mycotic abscess in the left cerebral hemiphere.

A left carotid angiogram disclosed a slight bow-shaped shift of the left anterior cerebral artery to the right; otherwise, there was no gross displacement and no obstruction of the main arterial branches. Subsequently, a ventriculography was done through bilateral postero-parietal burrholes in the face-down position under local anaesthesia. The dura mater was bulging on either side; no abscess was encountered with the exploring cannula. From both lateral ventricles there was free flow of fluid but only a few ml. were gained on either side. Ventri-

[1] Quoted from DIAMOND (1932), p. 1206.

cular catheters were inserted and secured to the skin. X-rays revealed a definite shift underneath the falx to the right with the right ventricle somewhat enlarged (Fig. 5). The overall impression from the plates was that of an enlarged bulk of the left hemisphere without any indication, however, of localised abscess formation.

Within three days a marked improvement was noticeable, the temperature and pulse rate gradually dropped and she was more alert and co-operative but still unable to talk; at times she was incontinent. The right arm remained paralysed; in the right leg, there was some return of active movements, and a nociceptive withdrawal reflex appeared; the ventricular catheters were then removed.

Three weeks later the temperature was down to normal and neurological improvement continued. Expressive speech was still difficult. Except for an intervening episode thought to be of embolic origin, she continued steadily improving on anticoagulants and high dosage of penicillin. When discharged after a four-months stay in hospital she was left with a slight facial paresis on the right and a weakness of her right arm and leg, the arm being more involved than the leg.

As to the nature of *the heart lesion*, the final assessment was this: most probably this was a rheumatic heart condition with gross mitral incompetence and a slight stenotic element, not so pronounced as to suggest surgery. There was nothing to indicate an auriculo-septal defect and subacute bacterial endocarditis was considered to be unlikely. An E.C.G. during reconvalescence showed sinus tachycardia and gross left ventricular strain in keeping with the diagnosis of mitral incompetence.

Comment. The conspicuous feature in this case was unilateral, left-sided, cerebral involvement as evinced both by the neurological findings and on air studies. Carotid angiography ruled out arterial obstruction (such as the one shown in Fig. 3) as well as gross abscess formation within the cerebral hemisphere involved. COURVILLE (1950) has emphasised the rarity of large brain abscess in cases of bacterial endocarditis. Also, the reversibility of the whole process as evidenced by slow, but definite, recovery suggests, in our case, absence of gross structural loss of brain tissue.

Since histological confirmation is lacking, it is difficult to classify the

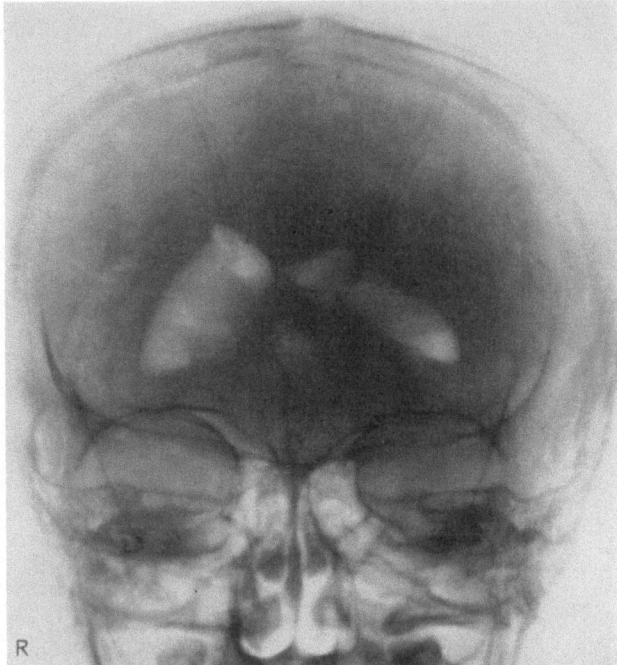

Fig. 5. Ventriculogram (p-a. view) in a child, aged 12, who took acutely ill with high temperature, confusion, neurological signs related to the left cerebral hemisphere, and high papilloedema. She had an enlarged heart and a systolic murmur. Rheumatic mitral incompetence was diagnosed and a mycotic cerebral abscess suspected but not confirmed. She recovered without operation. Note ventricular catheters in situ. (Case 0.3)

underlying process in terms of the various anatomo-pathological findings as mentioned above. It is rare for a bulky cerebral oedema to be confined to one hemisphere only, without a definite cause, either structural or vascular, involving the same hemisphere. There is general consensus, on the part of the morbid anatomists, as to the diffuse nature and multiplicity of cerebral involvement in cases of bacterial and rheumatic heart disease. On the other hand, it has long been thought that metastatic brain abscesses prefer the left cerebral hemisphere; although this is not substantiated by more recent findings, as will be discussed in Chapter D, nevertheless multiple embolism or, alternatively, a cortical thrombophlebitis seem a possibility, not too remote, to be considered in our case. The main issue, of course, was to rule out a brain abscess of surgical proportions; this was achieved by contrast methods and explorative needling, and confirmed by steadily progressing improvement.

5. Haemorrhage*

On the whole, it is rare for an intracranial haemorrhage, to be mistaken for intracranial suppuration because of the former's proneness to rapid development and its frequent

---

* Reference is made to the recent monographs by F. LOEW and S. WÜSTNER: Diagnose, Behandlung, Prognose der traumatischen Hämatome des Schädelinneren. Berlin-Wilmersdorf: Lange & Springer 1960. — W. KRAULAND: Über die Quellen des akuten und chronischen subduralen Hämatoms. Stuttgart: Georg Thieme 1961.

association with trauma and vascular disease. The converse is equally true. Among a total of 62 intracranial bleeds, cerebral and meningial, of traumatic origin, encountered up to 1958 (IRSIGLER, 1958) there were 20 extradural, 27 subdural, and 15 intracerebral clots; in only a few though important cases some of which will be mentioned presently, some kind of intracranial abscess formation was considered a possibility in differential diagnosis.

As to the *intracerebral clots:* Of surgical bearing are the bulky clots located within the subcortical white matter of one of the cerebral lobes. They frequently are of traumatic

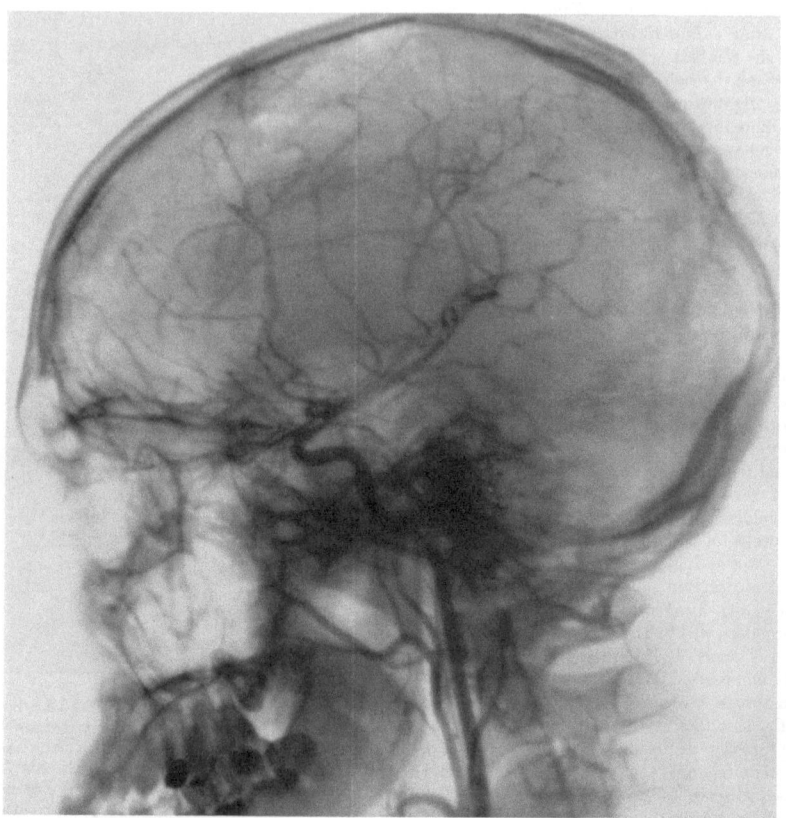

Fig. 6. Carotid arteriogram in a left-handed man, aged 22, with early type of intracerebral clot of traumatic origin in the right hemisphere. The clot was successfully aspirated through a single burrhole on the 6th day after injury. Site of clot is indicated by splaying - out of the ascending anterior branches of the sylvian group. The "arteriae insulares" of KRAYENBÜHL and RICHTER are compressed by the haematoma

etiology; so were half of the 41 cases reported by BUCKLEY and MCKINNEY in 1941. These bleeds show a certain tendency to be situated near the carrefour where the four cerebral lobes converge. Seven out of ten acute posttraumatic intracerebral clots collected by the present writer from the literature up to 1955 were within the temporal lobe (IRSIGLER, Thesis, 1955).

It is of interest to note that intracerebral haemorrhages associated with arterial hypertension and within the reach of the neurosurgeon owing to their subcortical location, reveal a similar predilection as was pointed out by the writer's Thesis on apoplectic cerebral haemorrhages. One of the first successfully removed clots in a hypertensive subject has been reported by GUTTMANN in 1936; it was confined to the right temporal lobe.

In many cases, however, the etiology remains obscure. WERNER (1954), in his study of 8 surgically treated cases of "spontaneous" subcortical haematomas from the Neuro-surgical Clinic in Zürich, was unable to establish the etiology in 7 of his patients. How broad the etiological range in so-called atypical or spontaneous cerebral haemorrhages really is becomes clear from the series by JEWESBURY.

The differential diagnosis from cerebral thrombosis and meningial bleed may be difficult or even impossible without ancillary surgical procedures, often a matter of emergency;

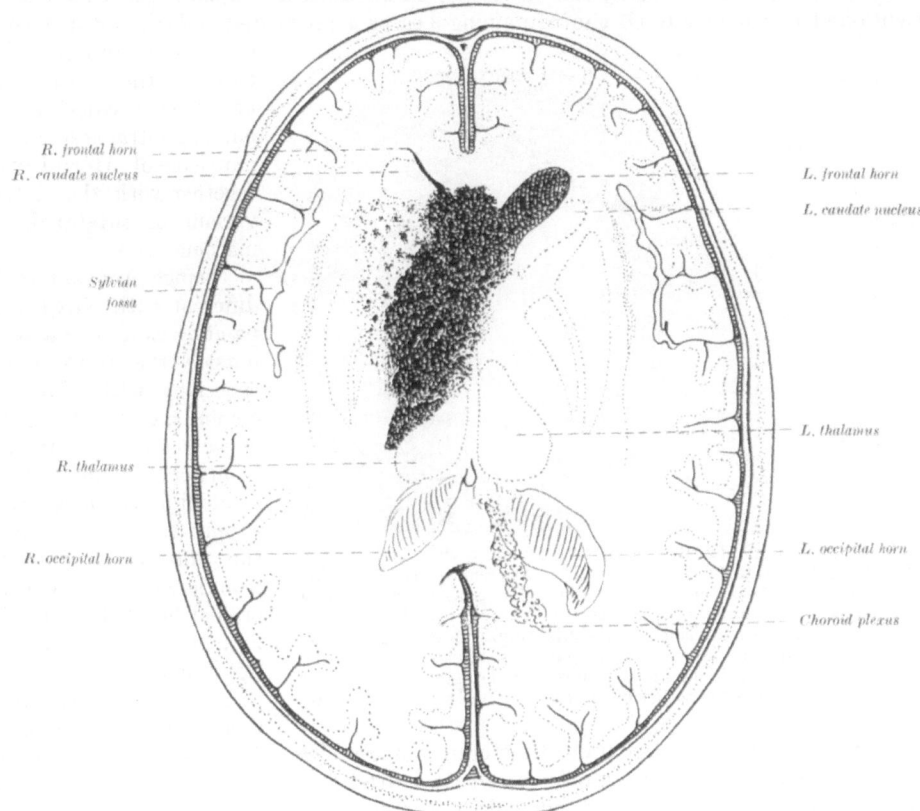

Fig. 7. Necropsy specimen. Horizontal section through the brain of a young adult who had been hit in his face and forehead 2 days prior to admission in deep coma. He died within a few hours. There was fracture of the left orbital roof and lamina cribriformis. Clinically, there were positive signs of brain stem damage right from the outset. Autopsy revealed haemorrhage into rostral part of basal ganglia and anterior limb of capsula interna on the right side; only parts of the caudate nucleus were spared. The clot extended across the midline into adjacent parts of the left frontal lobe with blood in the left anterior horn. It is significant that there was a sero-purulent leptomeningitis of rhinogenous origin on the base of the brain with pus and blood in the 4th ventricle

for, as a rule, these haemorrhages are ushered in by sudden migrainous headache, impaired consciousness, and neurological disability opposite to the side of hemicrania (WERNER); obviously, such a syndrome will make a cerebro-vascular accident most likely.

There is one exception, however, to this rule. Intracerebral haematomas adjacent to the ventricle may develop slowly and behave like a progressive expanding lesion; this is possibly consequent to an osmotic pressure gradient with slow fluid transfer from the ventricle (COURVILLE, 1950). A similar mechanism is probably effective also in chronic subdural haematomas. Only a few cases of this type of intracerebral haematoma up to now have been reported: by ROWBOTHAM and OGILVIE (1945), by the present author in his Thesis (1955) referred to above, and by COURVILLE in 1957. In none of these cases a suppurative lesion was suspected.

The acute traumatic intracerebral haemorrhage, be it subcortical and thus amenable to evacuation (Fig. 6), or be it located within the inaccessible parts of the brain i.e. the basal ganglia and the internal capsule (Fig. 7) as described by COURVILLE and BLOMQUIST, ANGRIST and MITCHELL, KRAULAND[1] and others, will hardly give rise to mistakes in diagnosis. Among 10 penetrating stabwounds of the head (Fig. 8) encountered during recent years by the present author, only one developed an intracranial suppuration; this case will be mentioned in Chapter B. Of the remaining 9 cases 4 recovered, 3 died, and in two the outcome is unknown. In two of the fatal cases necropsy revealed an expanding intracerebral haemorrhage of arterial origin together with the arterial variant of subdural haematoma.

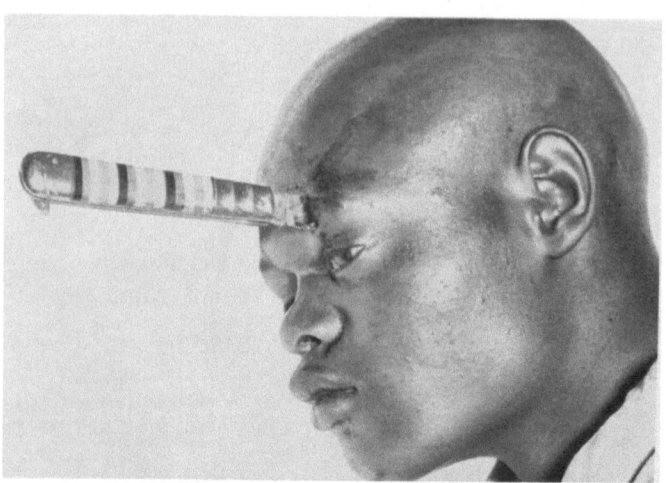

Fig. 8. This handy knife failed to enter the cranial cavities being stuck entirely within the bones of the base of skull. It was removed the following day after two attempts had been unsuccessful. The patient had not for a moment lost his consciousness after the assault. The only neurological signs were ptosis and slight exophthalmos (non-pulsating) with some restriction of ocular movements and insignificant impairment of vision on left. The optic fundi were normal. No infection developed and symptoms cleared up almost completely by the time of his discharge two weeks after admission

Things are somewhat different with chronic expanding clots beneath and outside the dura mater, especially with those becoming manifest late. Here as well as in patients with a history of penetrating head injury, intracranial suppuration must enter the differential diagnosis from late or interval intracranial bleed. Let us take first *the chronic subdural clot*. In clinical practice, it is a kind of proteus presenting in a kaleidoscopic fashion, under a variety of syndromes including brain abscess (Fig. 9). Most significant, to my experience, are headaches, frequently of an intermittent type, and a vacillating mental derangement that often is pictured, wrongly, as simple lowering of mental alertness correlated with supposed increase in intracranial pressure. However, it resembles much more what E. BLEULER has termed the "psych-organic syndrome" of which WALTHER-BÜEL lately has given a lucid analysis in his monograph (1951). This syndrome is closely related to BONHOEFFER's "exogenous reactive types" and to the amnesic-confabulatory syndrome of KORSAKOW.

In the previous history of patients with chronic subdural clots there is the well-known relation to trivial head-injuries of the blunt, non-penetrating type, and often forgotten because of their every-day character. Delirious and violent episodes, so frequent in chronic alcoholism, predispose, as it were, to repeated traumas of the minor type.

In pathogenesis, there is obviously a close association with episodes of low intracranial pressure which, as has been emphasized by SCHALTENBRAND and WOLFF, most probably are related to the shifting, fluctuating type of mental derangement mentioned above.

Mesencephalic involvement (Fig. 10), the clinical aspects of which have been stressed by NELSON in an important paper in 1942, has been found by the writer in the form of

[1] Quoted from PETERS (1951), p. 229.

Fig. 9. Ventriculogram (a-p. view) in an adult native who 14 days prior to admission had been hit over his head. 10 days after this incident he developed convulsions leaving him in coma and later confusion. He was referred to the neurosurgical unit with the diagnosis of frontal lobe abscess because of a fracture which was thought to involve the frontal sinus (it did not). A small amount of subdural blood was evacuated through a frontal burr hole on the 16th day after injury. Subsequently he improved mentally but developed bilateral papilloedema, rapidly progressing and amounting, on the right, to 4 diopters, with haemorrhages. Ventriculography now revealed a normal-sized but displaced ventricular system diagnostic of an expanding mass in the right temporal region. Following removal of a subdural clot $4^1/_2$ weeks after injury he again developed jacksonian fits on the left but recovered eventually fully. (On exposure, the brain and ventricular fluid had been found under considerable pressure in this case)

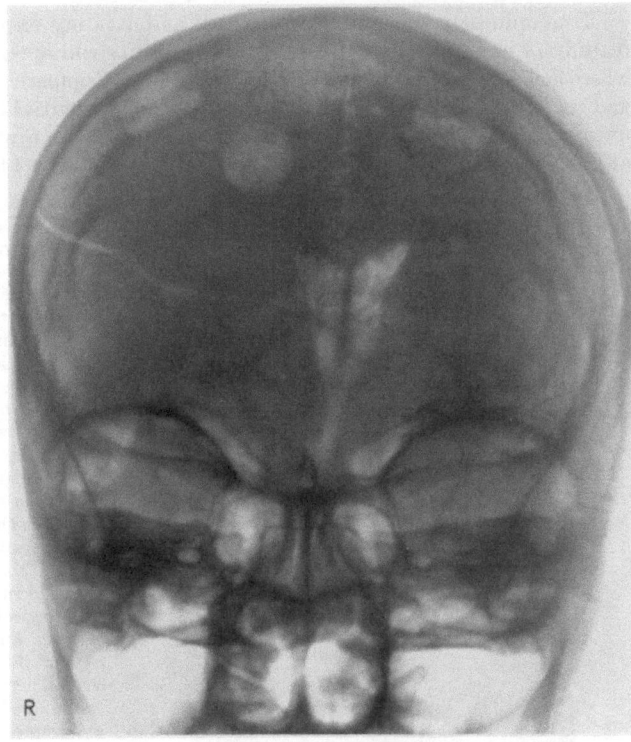

bulky haemorrhages apparent to the naked eye and obviously fatal in the cases concerned, in 10 out of 18 cases of acute flooding of the subdural spaces with blood following trauma. However, less extensive haemorrhages and ischaemic lesions within the mesencephalon may well be survived as has been shown by COURVILLE and AMYES (1952), and by WOLMAN (1953).

Fig. 10. Post mortem specimen. Left half of brain stem and cerebellum cut roughly in the sagittal plane, from a native adult who died 2 days following evacuation of acute subdural clot from right temporal fossa. Note haemorrhagic cavity in left quadrigeminal plate. Clinically: Coma throughout, hemiparesis on left, right pupil dilated and fixed, left pupil pin-point; bilateral Babinski's sign. Necropsy revealed no recurrent bleed but a bulky swelling of the right hemisphere extending into midbrain with considerable shift of the brain stem to left. Right lateral ventricle slit-like.

p . . . pons

(NB. A similar picture is to be found in a recent paper by R. LINDENBERG and E. FREYTAG, The Mechanism of Cerebral Contusions. A Pathologic-anatomic Study. Arch. Path. **69**, 440 (1960). In Fig. 18, the authors illustrate a "contusion haemorr-

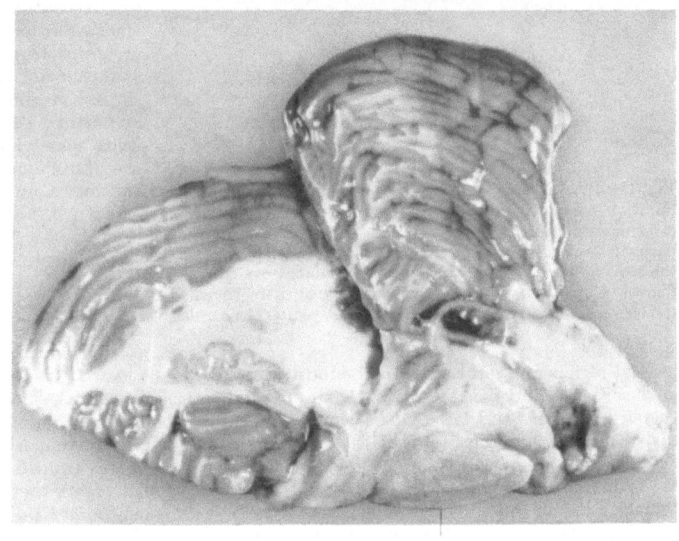

hage in the left brachium conjunctivum of upper pons" due to a shifting of the brain toward the tentorial opening with sudden temporary herniation.)[1]

---

[1] The reader is referred to the comprehensive monograph by H. W. PIA: Die Schädigung des Hirnstammes bei den raumfordernden Prozessen des Gehirns. Wien: Springer-Verlag 1957.

True epileptic seizures of any kind, as far as my experience goes, belong to the rare features of chronic subdural clot, and this is in striking contrast to the subdural empyema where jacksonian fits ceteris paribus are almost diagnostic as will be discussed in Chapter A, and consequently are a point of importance in differential diagnosis. I have seen jacksonian fits in patients with proved subdural haematoma only a few times (Fig. 9). One case met with at the Neurosurgical Clinic of the Charité in Berlin in 1944 is worth while mentioning here.

Case 0.4. Chronic subdural haematoma in a pregnant woman who developed convulsions. Eclampsia was diagnosed and pregnancy terminated. Later on the subdural clot was evacuated, and she recovered.

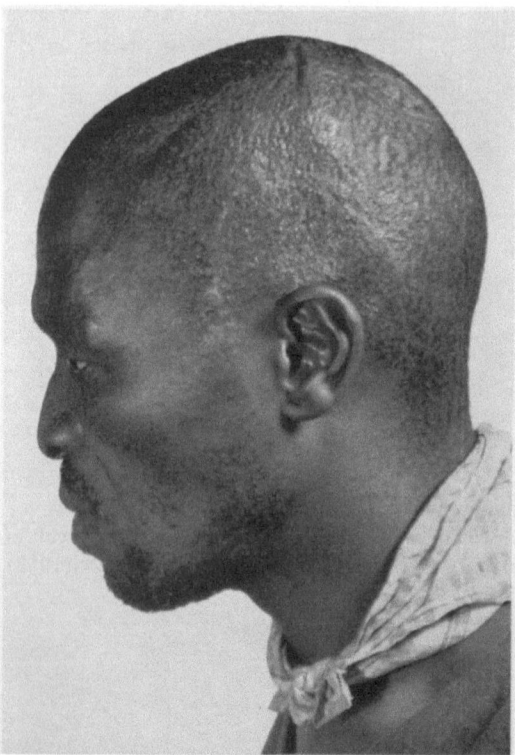

Fig. 11. In this man an epidural clot of about 2 weeks duration was evacuated through a small temporal flap (routine approach). There was a linear fracture of the left parietal bone and a septic wound of the scalp marking the site of injury. The above photo was taken 3 weeks following operation. A left carotid angiogram revealed the classical picture of a meningial bleed and thus ruled out a brain abscess

This was a woman who during the first trimester of pregnancy i. e. 9 months before admission, had a series of "small strokes" which left her with a transient weakness of the right half of her face. Six months later, at the beginning of the 9th month of her pregnancy, she had a similar attack and was admitted to a hospital where under the diagnosis of eclampsia the pregnancy was terminated. She was unconscious during this period, and, on coming round, noticed that her right arm and leg were paralysed and she was unable to talk. She then was transferred to the Neurosurgical Clinic of the Charité.

She was an attentive and bright woman with an aphasia mainly of the expressive type. When engaged in conversation, she made every attempt to express herself by means of speech as well as in writing. Fundoscopy revealed some venous congestion on the left and a normal fundus on the right side. There were no visual defects and no facial weakness. There was, in addition, a GERSTMANN's syndrome including astereognosis and (at least at times) body image agnosia of the right arm. She was unable to recognize familiar objects put into the palm of her right hand, and to perform finger movements necessary to carry out this task. Also deep sensation was impaired in the right hand and there was definite motor weakness of her right arm. Muscle power in the legs was equal, stance and walk normal.

Air studies showed no shift and a slight asymmetry of the lateral ventricles, the left one being somewhat larger. The subarachnoid spaces over both hemispheres contained a conspicuous amount of air. A tentative diagnosis of a diffuse vascular lesion was made, and cerebral thrombangitis von WINIWARTER-BUERGER was thought a possibility. To our surprise, a subsequent carotid angiogram disclosed a ventricular shift to the right and a crescent-shaped avascular area beneath the calvaria diagnostic of a chronic subdural clot. An osteoplastic flap was raised over the left fronto-parietal region and an encapsulated subdural haematoma removed in toto covering the greater part of the left hemisphere and being thickest over the medial parts near the sagittal sinus. The capsule contained several encysted pools of fluid blood. After removal of the membranes the hemisphere presented a conspicuous concavity and the convolutions exposed appeared small and shrunken, like in microgyria. To obliterate the dead space between the brain and dura mater the ventricle was tapped and refilled with saline whereupon the brain expanded sufficiently to allow dural closure without undue tension. A thin rubber wick was issued through a button hole and the wound closed in layers. Around the 3rd postoperative day the aphasia became more pronounced for a while without impairment of the receptive part of speech, however. After that, the patient made a good recovery. Follow-up studies could not been done in 1944.

Criticism. No doubt, the right side should have been explored, too. As this was not done no explanation can be offered for the lack of ventricular shift in the air encephalogram. Worth mentioning is the shrunken, as it were, "dehydrated" condition of the moulded hemisphere underlying the clot; in fact, COURVILLE and AMYES in 1952 expressed the view that in cases of chronic subdural haematoma moulding of the dorsolateral surface of the cerebral hemisphere beneath the clot is due to expression of its fluid content. This, it would appear, accounts for the widespread cortical damage to the left parietal and adjacent areas.

Turning now to *the extradural collections* we again expect those of late manifestation to arouse interest from the point of view of differential diagnosis.

Three cases of slow-developing type were seen among 20 patients with extradural haemorrhage reported by the author in 1958. One of these cases was complicated by an infected wound of approximately two weeks duration in the left parietal area. This man is illustrated in Fig. 11.

An impressive instance of such type of extradural clot has been related by ROWBOTHAM and WHALLEY in 1952; their clot was of four weeks standing and had grown to the remarkable size of 4 by 3 inches.

In the rare instances where the clot develops at an uncommon site it may even take longer before the diagnosis is made especially when signs of increasing pressure are mild or transient and papilloedema fails do develop. LINDGREN, in 1954, published a phlebogram quite similar to the one in Fig. 12 but, in his case, a fracture of the vault of the skull was present overlying the superior longitudinal sinus and no details were reported as to the history of this patient.

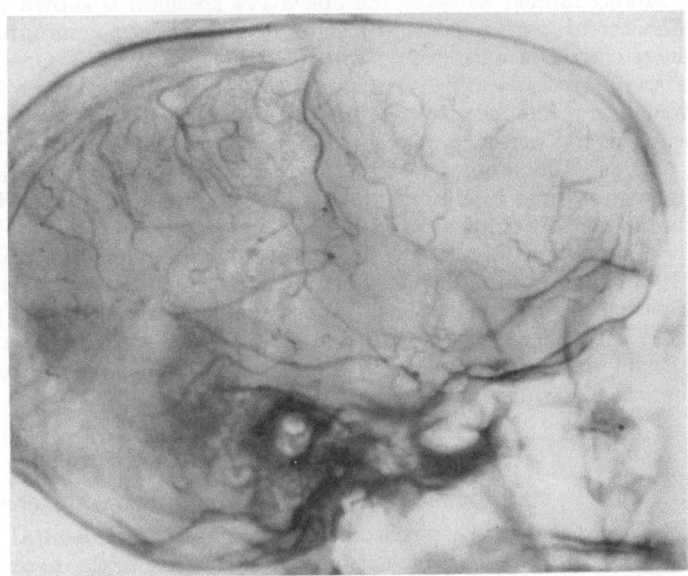

Fig. 12. Carotid phlebogram in man aged 26 who was picked up in the street inebriated and unconscious and with an abrasion over the right temple. He apparently had had a series of convulsions evinced by fresh bites in his tongue. He remained confused and with a right hemiparesis. A carotid angiogram was done 2 days after admission. No papilloedema developed but the patient was on artificial feeding for more than 4 weeks. A fluid extradural haematoma underlying the medial parts of the left hemisphere close to and beneath the sagittal sinus was washed out through a postero-parietal burrhole 5 weeks after admission. No clot was found on right. The patient recovered

In one of my own cases included in the series of 1958, a bilateral papilloedema developed suddenly on the 10th day of admission and a big extradural clot was then evacuated successfully from the middle fossa on the side of the dilated pupil. As this was a native boy of 8 years with a somewhat vague history and no obvious signs of trauma to the head, cerebral venous thrombosis, tuberculous meningitis, and even typhoid fever were considered in differential diagnosis.

A. The rhinogenous class

Classification of cases. There are 34 cases in this class with 11 fatalities giving a mortality rate of 33%.

This compares not unfavourably with the mortality rate of 34% in 44 brain abscesses of various etiology reported by BALLANTINE and SHEALY in 1959. SPERL and his co-workers reviewing their results in 60 patients with various kinds of brain abscess from the Mayo Clinic (1959), were able, with the combined use of antibiotics and surgery, to lower the overall mortality rate for brain abscess to 20%. Similarly, WEBER[1] in a recent paper

---

[1] G. WEBER: Traitement et résultats thérapeutiques des abscès cérébraux. Neuro-Chirurgie 6, 367 (1960).

reported a mortality rate of 21 % in a series of 57 acute and chronic cerebral abscesses treated by radical excision at the Zürich Clinic.

With regard to penetrating missile wounds, involving the paranasal air sinuses, which the author saw during the last war, only two have been included here and will be discussed in more detail in the Section on War Injuries; these are the cases 1.3 and 1.7.

The Rhinogenous Class has been divided into 4 Groups.

Four frontogenous brain abscesses form the first Group. One patient (case 1.1) died following radical excision; the operative specimen is shown in Fig. 13. Case 1.2 left the Clinic on his own request, with signs of streptococcal meningitis, 8 days after right frontal lobectomy. His case history will be discussed on p. 22. One patient whose case history starts on p. 21, eventually succumbed after a protracted period of intracranial suppuration and several unsuccessful surgical attempts. The last patient was discharged after radical excision and primary wound healing; the case history is reproduced on p. 20 et seq.

Group II encompasses 8 patients with frontal osteitis and POTT's "Puffy Tumour"; there were three fatalities in this Group, all three complicated by acute subdural empyema in the frontal region.

The traumatic cases are divided into two additional groups:

Group III contains 10 patients with fronto-basal fracture involving the paranasal sinuses but without dural leak; there were 5 fatalities in this group.

Finally, 12 cases are included in Group IV; these are the patients with fracture through the anterior air sinuses and with overt cerebro-spinal leak; none of them died, though in one the final outcome is not known.

I. The non-traumatic cases

1. Group I: Frontogenous abscess

The classical type which takes its origin from the frontal sinus is represented by the cases 1.5 and 1.2. Patients not infrequently come to the neurosurgeon after operation by the ear, nose and throat specialist, or while still being treated in their wards.

Maxillogenous abscesses of the brain are extremely rare, according to post mortem experiences at least (COURVILLE, 1950). They arise from osteomyelitis of the bony walls of HIGHMORE's antrum which nowadays becomes less common even in longstanding and disruptive lesions not subjected to operation. GURDJIAN and WEBSTER (1948a) include in their series a single case of a carcinoma originating from the cheek and orbit, associated with osteitis of the surrounding bone and eventually leading to a frontal lobe abscess; the patient recovered.

In the present series, there is one instance of brain abscess possibly consequent to maxillary empyema (case 1.12). This patient had, some months previously, a fracture to his maxilla and developed a sudden hemiplegia on the right side eight days before admission. 25 ml. of pus were aspirated from the left hemisphere. However, in the meantime, this patient also had developed a pleural empyema and it might well be that his brain abscess in fact was of metastatic origin. According to COURVILLE (1950) maxillogenous abscesses are likely to rupture into the tip of the temporal horn, a site from which one would hardly expect a hemiplegia.

Here, a few points regarding intracranial spread of infection will be discussed.

Routes of intracranial spread

a) By way of vascular channels

1. The *venous route* is probably the most common and was stressed by EAGLETON in 1922 following a remark by ATKINSON (1928, on p. 488). It is exemplified by three of the writer's cases. The infection is mediated by thrombophlebitis of the dural sinuses and/or cortical tributaries resulting in orthograde or retrograde extension of the infection above as well as below the tentorium cerebelli. The retrograde venous extension has been indi-

cated by PREYSING as early as 1901 (again following ATKINSON, 1928). It seems likely that many subdural abscesses, and especially those situated at a distance from the original site of infection, are initiated in this way. Thrombosis and thrombophlebitis of the superior longitudinal sinus and ascending frontal cortical veins play an important role in the spread of infection from the frontal sinus. In case 1.17 of the present series, a recent thrombus was found in the superior sagittal sinus at necropsy while several intramural abscesses were revealed under the microscope, scattered within the walls of the same sinus.

In the above series a tangle of thrombosed veins was found as an appendage to one end of the radically excised rhinogenous frontal abscess in two cases, each time giving the operative specimen a characteristic appearance; one of the cases is illustrated in Fig. 13.

The peculiar arrangement of encapsulated multiple or multilocular abscesses which are occasionally found to form a "chain" may also be related to the spread of infection creeping into the brain substance along vascular channels. It is at the site of these vascular "hili" that the abscess is likely to rupture during excision; this happened in case 1.2 (Fig. 15).

A good instance of this type of concatenated cerebellar abscesses has been presented by BOTTERELL and DRAKE (1952).

We shall return to the point of venous thrombosis in the Section on War Injuries when discussing case 1.7 there.

2. *The Emissaria.* The long-known importance of the emissary and diploic veins as portals of entry for infections from outside as well as from the accessory sinuses is mentioned here only in brief. Access into the anterior cranial fossa may be gained by infections

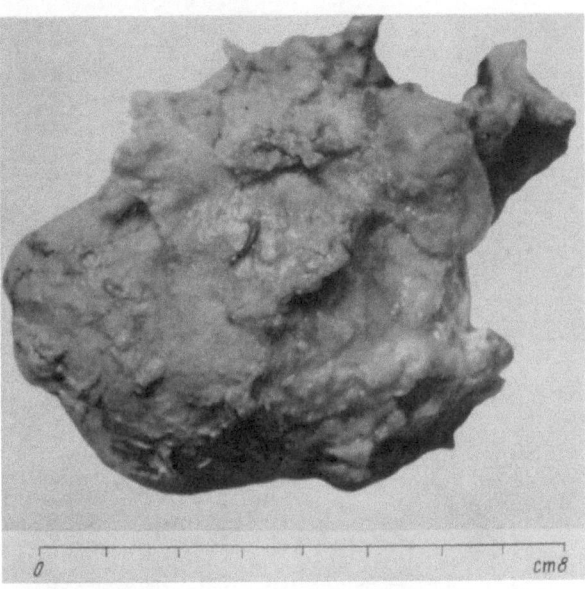

Fig. 13. Operative specimen of a radically excised rhinogenic frontal abscess (case 1.1). The appendage attached to the capsule on the right consists of a tangle of thrombosed veins draining into the cavernous sinus and deep cerebral veins. The patient survived the operation for only one week. Necropsy showed no residua of the abscess (1941)

via the v. diploica frontalis emerging at the upper margin of the orbit and communicating, on the one hand, with the naso-frontal and upper orbital veins, and with the angular and facial veins, on the other. The diploic venous channels may be compared to cross-roads draining into the superficial veins of the scalp as well as into the sinus durae matris over the convexity and at the base of the brain, the common pool there being the cavernous sinus. Into the dural sinuses "dip" the protrusions of the arachnoid villi. It will be noted also that there is a potential two-way direction of the blood flow within the diploic system, the flow being, under normal circumstances, cranio-petal; it may be reversed under pathological conditions such as cavernous sinus thrombosis, or carotid-cavernous fistula as was clearly demonstrated by WOLFF and SCHMID on carotid phlebograms.

3. *The arterial route* may well be a factor not yet fully realized. ATKINSON (1928) has drawn attention to intermediate arteriitis in the development of subcortical brain abscess of otogenic origin. Although he found it only in one out of 16 specimens this finding may have a more general bearing. The conspicuous transverse arrangement of the vascular channels within the white matter of the brain, emphasized by FISCHER and SCHEINKER, together with its paucity of blood supply as compared to the cerebral cortex, obviously is

closely related to the spread of cerebral oedema as well as to spread of infection within the brain substance.

b) Spread per continuitatem

In this case, the infection reaches the cranial cavity by involving, step by step, the contiguous structures en route to the brain producing in turn sub-aponeurotic cellulitis (case 1.16), frontal osteitis (case 1.5), extradural abscess (case 1.18), and subdural empyema (case 1.17).

Brain abscesses adjacent to osteomyelitis of the skull will be discussed in Chapter B.

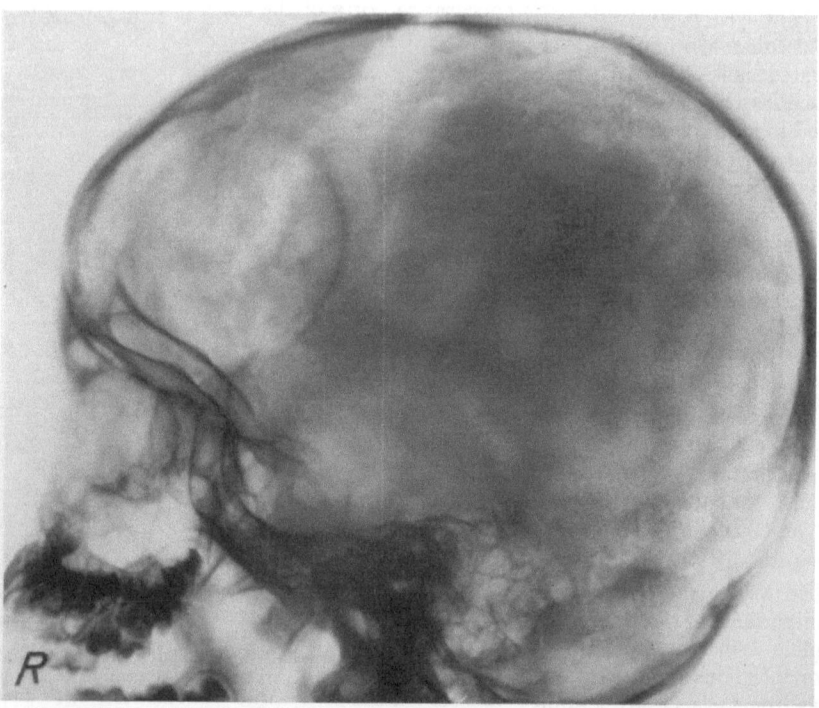

Fig. 14. Late frontal lobe abscess in a child who had struck her forehead nearly 3 months before acute signs and symptoms of increased intracranial pressure developed. Following a suggestion made by E. A. KAHN (1939) the abscess was visualised by thorotrast (Dr. M. J. JOUBERT) and subsequently successfully excised (Case 1.6)

In blunt, not-penetrating injuries to the forehead a sub-aponeurotic abscess in the frontal region may be a significant prelude to a late frontal lobe abscess. This is demonstrated by the following case 1.6.

Case 1.6. Right frontal lobe abscess in a child who had struck her forehead about 3 months previously. Involvement of the fronto-basal region has not been established beyond doubt; however, a subaponeurotic abscess over the forehead had been evacuated 4 weeks prior to radical excision of the brain abscess. Recovery.

This was a girl of 5 years who had struck her forehead 2 months before she was admitted with a subapo-neurotic abscess in the right frontal region. This abscess was incised. At the same time, a right frontal lobe abscess was suspected and therefore the brain explored with a brain cannula (Dr. M. J. JOUBERT).. No abscess was found. About 4 weeks later, she was readmitted with signs of rapidly increasing intracranial pressure. Reexploration now revealed a huge, well-encapsulated abscess in the right frontal lobe which subsequently was visualised with colloidal thorium dioxide (thorotrast) as shown in Fig. 14 X-rays showed, in addition, marked separation of the coronal suture and a silver-beaten calvaria. Subsequently, the abscess was excised in toto. It had a dense capsule and was the size of a hen's egg. It lay in the subcortical white matter necessitating decapping of the right frontal lobe. The impression was that of a multilocular abscess. The dura mater was closed and sprinkled with achromycin powder. The thin bone was reinserted and the flap resutured without drain in two layers. She recovered rapidly and permanently.

Comment. As was mentioned in the introductory section (p. 6) the differential diagnosis from a neuroblastoma of the skull was well to be kept in mind in this case. The clue was given by the preceding trauma; the subaponeurotic abscess at the site of injury provided the intermediary link in the development of events.

c) The straightforward avenue

The straightforward avenue from the frontal, ethmoid and sphenoid cavities is mainly seen in traumatic cases and in missile wounds of the fronto-orbital region. It leads straight into the subarachnoid pools at the base of the brain with the infection resulting in a "primary" basal leptomeningitis which develops during the very first days after injury. CAIRNS, CALVERT, DANIEL, and NORTHCROFT (1947) have termed it "meningitis of immediate or very early onset". Infection along this route is seldom followed by abscess formation (COURVILLE, 1950). It will be more fully discussed in the section on fronto-basal injuries.

This chapter is concluded by two representative case histories of rhinogenic frontal abscess. From their discussion some points of clinical importance will emerge to round off the theoretical exposé.

Case 1.5. Man, aged 20. Frontal osteitis following radical operation for frontal sinus infection. Dura mater incised by the ENT. specialist. Protracted course resulting in brain herniation and right frontal abscess. Aspiration and drainage of the abscess. Death after a lengthy period of intracranial suppuration.

A soldier, aged 20, had some 4 months previously an operation performed on his frontal sinus by the otologist. No details were available. An osteomyelitis of the frontal bone was found or perhaps developed soon after the Killian procedure, and a large trephine opening was made in the region of the glabella. The patient went on complaining of severe headache and insomnia and finally, signs of raised intracranial pressure became apparent.

On admission, there was a cerebral fungus size of a golf ball in the region of the frontal sinus. It was covered with granulations and around its base, the fungus was rather firmly attached to the skin edges and in part covered by them. There was a surgical scar 12 cm in length just above the eye brows. The soft tissues overlying the trephine opening were under high tension and bulging. A second operative scar ran parallel to the one mentioned within the hair line; obviously this was a relaxation incision. The X-rays showed a big roundish defect in the middle of the frontal bone, there were no residua of the frontal sinus left.

The patient was drowsy but responsive and well orientated. Both optic discs were choked. The pupils were equal and reacted to light. No neck rigidity was noted. A complete hemiparesis on the left side was present including the left half of the face. The tone and the tendon reflexes in the left arm and leg were increased and the plantar response was extensor on the left side.

Lumbar puncture revealed a clear and colourless fluid under increased pressure with marked pleocytosis.

The diagnosis of a right frontal abscess was confirmed by ventriculography.

Under local anaesthesia, a skin-galea flap was turned down in the right frontal region and the dura incised around the neck of the cerebral herniation. At a depth of about 8 cm an abscess was struck with the brain cannula and approximately 10 ccm. of thick, yellow, odourless pus were aspirated. The previous trephine opening was now enlarged and with the diathermy needle the abscess cavity laid open. An additional 30 to 35 ccm. of pus were removed by suction. The inner surface of the pyogenic membrane was smooth and shiny. A rubber tube was inserted into the abscess cavity and anchored to the edge of the dura mater. The skin flap was resutured and a compression dressing was applied. The patient was subsequently transferred to a military hospital; no details of the postoperative course are available. It is known however that he died after several weeks of intracranial suppuration.

Comment. This patient developed after a KILLIAN procedure an osteomyelitis of the adjacent frontal bone which necessitated radical removal of the whole of the frontal sinus including the surrounding bone. Nothing is known with regard to involvement of the dura mater and the subdural structures at the time when this trephine opening was made. During a prolonged course of several months and in spite of sulfonamide therapy a cerebral fungus of considerable size developed and signs of intradural infection became apparent. A purulent collection behind the cerebral herniation resulted in a deep abscess within the right frontal lobe of the brain. Incision and drainage of this abscess proved inadequate obviously because of the brain fungus occluding the trephine opening in the frontal bone.

It can hardly be doubted that a better approach would have been turning down a frontal osteoplastic flap followed by radical excision of the right frontal lobe including the well-encapsulated abscess and redundant cerebral hernia. However, it must be realized that in 1941 no antibiotics were yet available and even the sulphonamide treatment in this case possibly was inadequate. In addition, it would appear sound practice, in frontal osteitis complicating frontal sinus infection, if it is deemed necessary to incise the dura mater, to seek neurosurgical advice in time in order to search for and eliminate an intradural lesion such as subdural empyema or brain abscess before a brain fungus with its deleterious effects develops.

Case 1.2. Boy of 17. Multilocular rhinogenous frontal abscess developing some eight weeks after evacuation of an abscess in the right upper lid. Rupture during excision of the right frontal lobe followed by streptoccocal meningitis.

In this patient a subcutaneous abscess in the right upper eye-lid had been incised and evacuated some eight weeks before admission. Subsequently, the patient complained of headache and failing vision, and became eventually progressively drowsy. When seen in the ward, he had high papilloedema on both sides, a markedly increased sedimentation rate, and the X-rays of the skull disclosed the frontal sinus densely shadowed with lack of detail of its outlines. Neurologically, no localising signs were present. In search for a right frontal abscess, two burr holes were made over the right frontal and rolandic areas. However, neither the ventricle, nor an abscess was struck. The following day an hemiplegia was noticed on the left side; a right carotid angiogram now revealed a mass near the frontal pole.

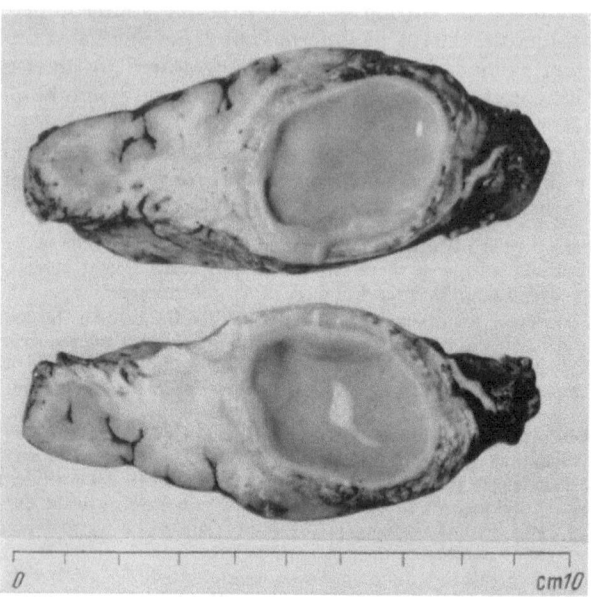

An osteoplastic frontal flap was turned down on the right with the incision crossing the midline to the left. The tense dura mater was incised and reflected. The leptomeninges over the surface were cloudy and with a white-yellowish tint. The dura mater was found adherent to the brain around the frontal pole. After plugging the subdural spaces with cotton wool, a frontal lobectomy was started. When, in the process of excision, the frontal pole was being mobilised and lifted up from the base, a sudden gush of creamy, yellow pus welled up from the depth and was carefully sucked off. The structures on the base of the brain then became accessable. The right anterior cerebral artery was found closely attached to the pyogenic membrane forming the capsule of a brain abscess which (in the operative specimen) had the size of a peach. The artery was severed between silver clips. Another, somewhat smaller, abscess was found occupying the frontal pole itself. It was surrounded by a thin membrane and it was at this site that the abscess had ruptured at the beginning of the excision. Lobectomy now was completed and resulted in exposing

Fig. 15. Operative specimen of a rhinogenous frontal lobe abscess which was excised some 8 weeks after evacuation of a subcutaneous abscess of the right upper eyelid. X-ray films showed opacity of the frontal sinus. Note thick pyogenic membrane surrounding the pent-up pus within the brain tissue. Another, smaller abscess which is not visible in the picture, ruptured during excision giving rise to streptococcal meningitis. (Case 1.2)

a healthy-looking, shiny dura mater covering the floor of the right anterior fossa. There was a tiny tear in the ependyma of the right anterior horn. The dura was closed tightly without a drain. The wound was resutured in layers. The operative specimen is shown in Fig. 15.

Within the ensuing 8 days the patient developed, despite high dosage of sulphonamides, a meningitis and from the lumbar fluid haemolytic streptococci were cultured. Pus escaped through the scalp incision. At the request of his parents the boy was discharged home in poor condition.

Comment. This was a therapeutic rather than a diagnostic problem, since the larval stage of a frontal osteitis which complicated frontal sinus infection and resulted in a dependent abscess of the right upper eye lid, provided the clue to the diagnosis of a right frontal abscess of rhinogenic origin. Explorative needling for the abscess resulted in hemiplegia which obviously was due to spreading cerebral oedema. Carotid angiography is preferable as a diagnostic procedure (WEBER, 1957), and confirmed, in this case, the presence of a mass in the right frontal lobe near the midline. It should be remembered, and it was shown clearly on the operating table in the case under discussion, that a frontogenic abscess will be located near the floor of the anterior fossa and in the frontal pole rather than near the convexity of the brain. The latter type appears more often associated with thrombophlebitis of the cortical veins and subdural empyema (COURVILLE, 1950). Multiplicity or multilocular growth of frontal abscesses of rhinogenic origin has to be reckoned with in planning and performing radical excision. In the above case, in spite of a history of some 8 weeks duration and careful handling during operation, one of the abscesses near the base was ruptured. Nowadays, with powerful antibiotics available, such rupture would hardly influence the prognosis and outcome. Sulphonamides such as were available in 1942 failed to prevent a fatal meningitis which, in the above case, possibly was due to direct infection of the anterior horn of the lateral ventricle.

2. Group II: Frontal osteitis and Pott's "Puffy Tumour"; subdural empyema in the frontal region

The two cases discussed in the foregoing section have already demonstrated clearly the intermediate rôle played by infectious osteitis, focal or spreading, of the frontal bone in the development of intracranial suppuration though, it must be admitted, in case 1.2, infection of the structures surrounding the frontal sinus could be inferred only from the history indicating cellulitis and abscess formation in the loose tissues around the right eye which preceded the clinical symptoms of a frontogenous brain abscess by some 8 weeks.

A brawny, often pitting, oedema of the scalp on the forehead is a characteristic sign of frontal osteitis consequent to infection of the frontal sinus or to local trauma to the skull. It is this type of oedema frequently giving, on palpation, the impression of fluctuation or actually fluctuant due to presence of pus in the sub-aponeurotic layer, which was described by PERCIVAL POTT in 1760 and after him called "POTT's Puffy Tumour". POTT found it in cases of extradural abscess complicating osteomyelitis arising from frontal sinus infection or consequent to fracture of the cranial vault (BOYD).

Table 1. POTT's *puffy tumour and related lesions*

Case no. age in ()	POTT's tumour	Intracranial suppuration	Outcome
1.16 (14)	Orbital cellulitis and subapo-neurotic abscess	none X-rays: mottled bone	Incision, drainage. Recovered
1.17 (13)	Pitting oedema	Subdural empyema X-rays: frontal sinus opaque[1]	Trephine openings. Died within 4 days
1.18 (37)	Fluctuant oedema	Extradural abscess X-rays: mottled bone[1]	Evacuation. Recovered
1.19 (12)	Fluctuant oedema	none X-rays negative	Incision. Recovered
1.20 (15)	Peri-orbital oedema & fluctuation (ptosis, exophthalmos, chemosis)	none X-rays: rarification ?	Spontaneous evacuation. Recovered
1.21 (10)	Fluctuant oedema	Cavernous sinus thrombosis. X-rays: pan-sinusitis with fluid levels; translucency ?[1]	Antibiotics; recovered without operation
1.22 (9 months)	Fluctuant oedema of forehead, descending to involve both eyes	H.influenza meningitis, sub-dural empyema. X-rays: sepa-rated sutures, frontal trans-lucency	Trephining and evacuation; antibiotics. Died after 5 weeks
1.23 (12)	none	Subdural empyema; no X-rays	Trephining, antibiotics. Died within 2 days
1.2 (17)	Abscess in right upper eyelid evacuated	Right frontal lobe abscess. X-rays: frontal sinus opaque[1]	Rupture during excision; meningitis
1.5 (20)	Frontal osteomyelitis contigu-ous to frontal sinus infection; dura incised by the aural surgeon	left frontal lobe abscess behind huge cerebral fungus[1]	Abscess drained; died after protracted course

In the present monograph 8 cases have been included as closely related to frontal osteitis although, it will be noted from Table 1, in some of the patients, infection of the bone was present in a larval stage only, such as suggested by POTT's oedema or inferred from previous history. A POTT's puffy tumour was absent only in one case, a subdural empyema of cryptogenic (metastatic?) origin (case 1.23).

In the synoptic Table 1 featuring the points of interest are included also the two frontogenous abscesses already referred to in the previous section dealing with rhinogenous brain abscesses.

Before turning to the conclusions derived from the data in Table 1 the following case histories will serve to picture some of the more important features of this kind of lesion.

---

[1] Pathogenetic relation to frontal sinus infection definitely established.

Case 1.18 may be considered as the classical type of POTT's puffy tumour associated with recurrent exacerbation of frontal sinus suppuration which, in this patient, dated back for many years.

Case 1.18. African male, aged 37. Repeated attacks of purulent frontal sinusitis followed by POTT's tumour with throbbing pain over the forehead. Evacuation of extradural frontal abscess by craniectomy. Recovery.

This man had suffered from recurrent attacks of frontal sinus empyema and fair quantities of pus were removed by the aural surgeon on several occasions. On admission in July, 1957, his only complaints were throbbing pain in his forehead and intermittent purulent discharge from the nose. On questioning it was found that his history dated back to 1939 when he had a first attack of this kind. The scalp over both frontal regions

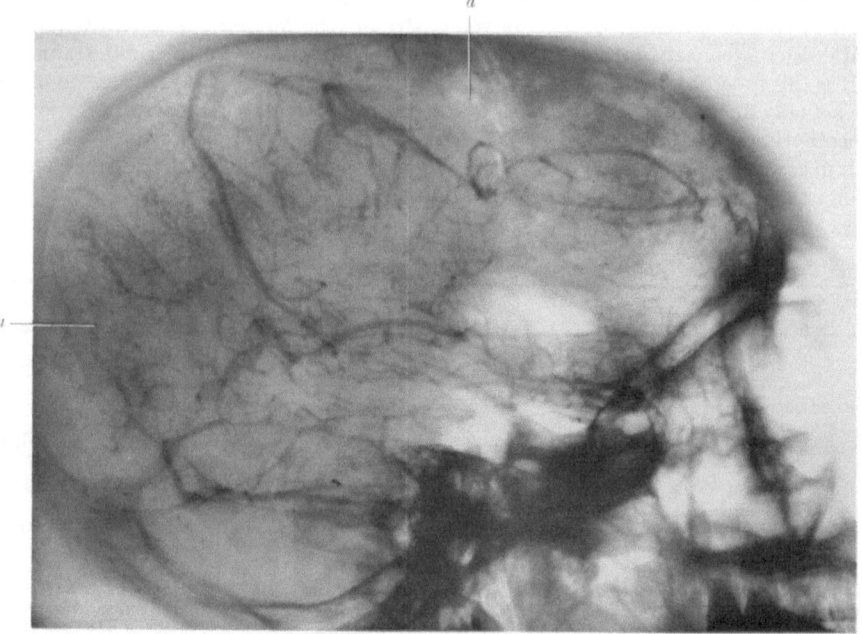

Fig. 16. Carotid angiogram (venous phase, lateral view) in a man from whom subsequently an extradural abscess in the frontal region was evacuated successfully after repeated attacks, dating back for many years, of frontal sinusitis attended to by the aural surgeon. At the time when the extradural abscess was removed exploration of the frontal sinus was negative. The prominent signs were Pott's tumour and throbbing pain over the forehead. Note chronic sclerosing osteitis of the frontal squama and displacement of the superior sagittal sinus together with group of ascendent frontal veins caused by the abscess. Both anterior horns contain air (from the air encephalogram); they are symmetrically displaced too. (Case 1.18) a .. angulus venosus indicating foramen of MONRO

was of a brawny, fluctuant consistence. Neurological examination revealed no abnormalities. X-rays disclosed opacity over the whole frontal sinus and a much thickened frontal squama of mottled appearance indicating chronic sclerosing osteitis. After air insufflation through the cisternal route both anterior horns were well visualised on the plates and both were displaced downwards. Likewise, a carotid angiogram evinced a significant displacement (Fig. 16). A bifrontal osteoplastic flap, concealed behind the hairline, was raised and a quadrangular piece of ivory bone excised underneath which a fairly big extradural abscess, surrounded by a smooth pyogenic membrane was found. More than 1 fluid ounce of thick pus was evacuated in one stage. Although the pyogenic membrane could be removed in part only, the wound healed per primary intention under penicillin and streptomycin, administered systemically as well as locally through thin rubber tubes. The man was restored to full working capacity within 4 weeks from the operation and has remained well since 1957.

Comment. There are several points requiring commenting in this case.

The frontal bone was sclerosed throughout and truly ivory both the outer and inner table being thickened. This is understandable considering the length of previous history. In addition, on excising the bone flap it was found that the bone was bloodless indicating necrosis. We did not trouble to remove completely the avascularized bone as suggested by ADSON and HEMPSTEAD (1937) at a time when modern chemotherapy was still at its infancy.

In doing the first trephine opening a thin tensile membrane was struck and at once perforated with the burr; it represented the pyogenic membrane surrounding the extradural abscess but, at first sight, gave the impression that we were dealing with a subdural empyema. This thin pyogenic membrane adhered to the inner surface of the excised bone. The yellow, creamy pus pent-up within the capsule had a tinge of foul smell and gram-negative bacilli of the coli-type were cultured from it. It is debatable whether this should be interpreted in favour of a metastatic rather than a frontogenic etiology.

As has been emphasized by ADSON and HEMPSTEAD the frontal sinus should be explored carefully at the time of craniotomy by removing its posterior wall. In the above case, this exploration was done concurrently by the ear, nose and throat specialist, through the old scar above the right eye; no pus was found, however, and the underlying dura was also clean. This was the more remarkable because, some months previously, a fair amount of pus had been removed from the frontal sinus by the KILLIAN approach. Moreover, at the time of craniectomy careful search for a communication between the abscess and the frontal sinus — or what was left of it — was negative. This and a local injury to his forehead, which the patient admitted to have suffered "many years ago," and which had left him with a curved scar in the region of the bregma, leave the question of traumatic origin of the frontal osteitis in this case somewhat unsettled.

To illustrate the difficulties which may arise in differential diagnosis the following two case histories, so different in their course and outcome, are briefly summarized here.

Case 1.21. POTT's tumour in acute pan-sinusitis, complicated by signs indicative of cavernous sinus thrombosis. Expectant treatment. Recovery under chemotherapy.

A girl of 10 fell acutely ill with pyrexia and vomiting. There was a perforation of the left ear drum and well marked fluctuant oedema of the forehead spreading from the glabella on either side upwards. X-rays of the skull indicated fluid levels within both maxillary antra. While on the X-ray table the patient developed epileptic convulsions requiring intravenous barbiturates. In the lumbar fluid there were 25 polymorphonuclears and 2 lymphocytes to the cmm. Within the ensuing few days a slight exophthalmos developed on the right together with ptosis of the right upper eye-lid and a slight squint due to weakness of the right internal rectus muscle. There was a query sensory loss over the supraorbital area; the left optic disc was possibly choked while the right papilla was normal. A paresis of the 6th nerve on the right could not be established beyond doubt. There was no neck rigidity and no localising signs apart from those mentioned, except for a query extensor plantar response on the left. Under heavy dosage of antibiotics, including ilotocin, the temperature settled down while the fluctuation over the forehead became still more pronounced. There was alo puffiness of the right temple and orbital region. Incision of a subaponeurotic abscess on the forehead was eventually deferred because, by then, the condition rapidly improved. Repeated X-rays of the skull revealed a middle-sized frontal sinus the boundaries of which were indistinct on the right and there was an adjacent area of increased translucency in the frontal bone. The patient recovered fully. Radiological examination on discharge from the hospital revealed an opaque frontal sinus, a normal frontal bone and normal maxillary antra.

Case 1.23. Haematogenous (?) subdural abscess in an African female of 12. Admission diagnosis: Tuberculous meningitis. Jacksonian epilepsy. Pleocytosis in the lumbar fluid. Frontal trephine openings. Death within two days of admission.

The girl was admitted while unconscious; no history was available. A tuberculous meningitis was suspected. Lumbar taps on several occasions revealed a clear and colourless fluid with 154 polymorphonuclears and 34 lymphocytes while sugar and chlorides were both within normal range. On examination she was in deep coma, incontinent, and not responding to painful stimulation. There was pronounced neck rigidity and a remittent temperature reaching at peaks 103° F. Incoordinate movements of the eyes as well as persistent twitchings on the entire left side of her body were noticed. Fundoscopy revealed venous congestion but no choroidal tubercles. There was a query left facial weakness, the limbs were flaccid with tendon reflexes hardly elicitable. There was a doubtful up-going toe on the left. From 2 frontal burr holes a big subdural empyema was encountered on the right and thick pus evacuated from which haemolytic streptococci were cultured. Attempts were made to establish subdural drainage. On repeated penicillin instillations the impression was gained that the pus was too thick for drainage and the subdural space becoming obliterated. She died within two days of admission. Necropsy (Dr. W. I. PEPLER) revealed a subdural abscess with concomitant leptomeningitis and endarteritis within the underlying cerebral tissue. No thrombosis of the dural sinuses was present in the parts examined.

In the following case a POTT's tumour, possibly related to paranasal sinus infection, was indicative of a fulminating frontal osteitis and a fatal bilateral subdural empyema. The etiology of infection in this patient has not been established beyond doubt, and will be discussed in the light of necropsy findings at the close of the case history.

Case 1.17. African boy, aged 13, POTT's puffy tumour of acute onset and fulminating course. Admission diagnosis: Cavernous sinus thrombosis. Herpetic eruption of the upper lip. Opacity of frontal sinus on the X-rays. Exploration of the frontal sinus. Bilateral frontal burr holes. Bilateral subdural empyema, encapsulated and completely removed on the left. Temporary improvement. Status epilepticus. Hemiplegia on left. Death 4 days after admission. Autopsy: Thrombosis of superior sagittal sinus with intramural abscesses. Purulent leptomeningitis.

This boy was admitted as an emergency case. He had suddenly taken ill 4 days previously with headache and a puffy swelling on his forehead, pyrexia, stiff neck, and progressive drowsiness. A cavernous sinus thrombosis was suspected. On examination he was stuporous with amorphous restlessness of all limbs. His temperature was 104° F. There was pronounced neck rigor; passive movements of his head seemed to be very painful. There was a pitting oedema of the scalp occupying the region of the glabella. There was no periorbital oedema and no chemosis. The pupils were middle-sized and reacting to light. Fundoscopy was difficult but the right papilla seemed to be congested, with sharp edges; the periphery of the left fundus appeared normal. There was an herpetic eruption of the upper lip. The ear drums were normal. There were no other neurological abnormalities except for an equivocal extensor response on the right. The plain X-rays of the skull revealed some haziness of the frontal sinus. The lumbar fluid was under raised pressure and clear. Under the microscope pneumococci (?) were found, the culture was negative. The day after admission the E.N.T. surgeon made an incision above the left eye and nibbled away some bone. He found a single ethmoid cell overlying the left orbit. No pus was encountered. The dura was not exposed, two rubber slivers were inserted. The same day the patient developed a complete left-sided hemiplegia. The fundi were still within normal. In spite of massive antibiotics the patient's temperature remained high and the doughy oedema over the frontal bone became more pronounced. An exploratory trephine opening was made now in the left temporo-parietal region and an encapsulated subdural abscess was encountered. A fair amount of yellow pus and mucoid debris was evacuated from within a thin pyogenic membrane which subsequently was removed gently, uncovering the leptomeninges which appeared somewhat inflamed; no pus, however, was present within the pia-arachnoid. A thin rubber catheter was inserted subdurally. Another burr hole was then made over the right frontal area and the dura exposed. It had a yellowish tinge; again, a subdural empyema was found and dealt with in a similar way as on the opposite side. On the right, however, the capsule adhered more firmly to the brain surface so as to prevent its complete removal. Two rubber drains were inserted and the subdural space subsequently irrigated with penicillin solutions.

The patient seemed to come slightly more to the surface, but the following day he developed jacksonian fits involving the left side of his body, and gradually merging into a status epilepticus. He succumbed within 4 days of admission, i.e. 8 days from the onset of his illness.

The important findings on the post mortem table were: Subaponeurotic abscess covering the greater part of the frontal bone, more so on the left, and extending behind the coronal suture. In both parieto-occipital regions, the galea aponeurotica showed patchy discolouration indicating necroses. No signs of previous trauma to the epicranium were found on careful examination. The frontal squama beneath the abscess had a conspicuous yellowish tinge indicating recent purulent *osteomyelitis*. After reflecting the dura mater the anterior ²/₃ of the right cerebral hemisphere were found covered with a pyogenic membrane of intense yellow colour and several mms. in thickness, firmly attached, at places, to the brain surface. No subdural pus or membrane was found on the left side. There was recent thrombosis of the superior longitudinal sinus extending into the right lateral and sigmoid sinuses. No leptomeningitis, cortical thrombophlebitis nor brain abscess were present to the naked eye. The paranasal sinuses and the right petrous bone were carefully searched for signs of infection. No pathology was found there, also the mucosal lining of the sphenoid sinus was intact. Histology (Dr. W. J. PEPLER) confirmed recent thrombosis of the superior sagittal sinus in the wall of which several intramural abscesses were found.

Comment. To the post mortem examiner the etiology of the frontal osteitis remained obscure. There was little to indicate spread of infection from the paranasal sinuses or from a distant suppurative lesion. There were no unequivocal signs of a previous head trauma either. Subdural clots of traumatic origin especially those following penetrating bullet wounds may give rise to purulent collections presenting as true subdural empyemas (NOETZEL[1]; TÖNNIS, 1945). Sagittal sinus thrombosis has been found not infrequently in large necropsy series of frontal subdural abscess, as a concomitant lesion indicating the route by which infection gained access to the intracranial structures (COURVILLE, 1944).

Subdural empyema following purulent meningitis has been described by SPITZ, POLLAK and ANGRIST[2]. On the whole, this sequence of events is uncommon except, perhaps, in the very young age group. KAHN (1955) gave an example of successful treatment by drainage and penicillin instillations of a child of 2¹/₂ years with a right-sided subdural abscess following haemophilus influenzae meningitis. The case which follows was seen in consultation by the author in 1958.

Case 1.22. H.influenzae meningitis in a baby of 9 months, followed by POTT's puffy tumour, subaponeurotic abscess and a huge subdural empyema over the right cerebral hemisphere. Despite catheter drainage and chemotherapy death occurred 5 weeks after admission.

A baby, aged 9 months, was admitted with signs of meningitis. The lumbar fluid was turbid, with marked pleocytosis, mainly polymorphonuclears. H. influenzae was isolated from the fluid. The temperature settled but within 10 days of admission a fluctuating swelling appeared over the forehead and the lumbar fluid remained purulent. X-rays of the skull revealed separated sutures and a query area of increased translucency in the right frontal bone close to the midline. The swelling gradually extended downward and forward to involve the eye-lids and the upper part of the face.

---

[1] H. NOETZEL's paper appeared in Zbl. Path. **81**, 3 (1943).
[2] Quoted from WEBER, G. (1957), pp. 79 and 184.

A frontal flap was raised and, after evacuation of a subaponeurotic abscess, thick pus was seen exuding from beneath the frontal bone through the metopic suture. Two trephine openings were then placed close to the sagittal sinus. The bone there was soft and pulpy. On the left side the dura mater was under tension but no pus was found neither above nor beneath it. On the right, however, an enormous amount of pus was recovered from beneath the dura mater and from an additional burr hole in the right parietal region. The subdural empyema was found to extend practically over the whole of the right hemisphere. Catheter drainage and instillations with chloromycetin were instituted. Culture from the subdural pus proved sterile, probably due to foregoing chemotherapy. The infant improved only for a while and died 5 weeks after admission. Throughout the course of the illness no convulsions of any kind were noticed. Necropsy was not granted.

Finally, the following two case histories will illustrate the comparatively mild course taken, at times, by infection of the frontal bone and the overlying structures of the epicranium closely related, anatomically and clinically, to the accessory sinuses; it is significant that such cases often are referred by the ophthalmologist or the ENT-specialist for assessment as to a possible intracranial suppuration.

Case 1.16. A native boy of 14 was admitted to the E.N.T. ward under the tentative diagnosis of intraorbital cellulitis and cavernous sinus thrombosis. There was fluctuating temperature and marked protrusion of the right eye. Skull X-rays revealed wide-spread patchy erosion of the frontal bone giving it a significant mottled appearance. Small cuts were made first in the upper lids of both eyes, and glove drains inserted. In addition, two linear scalp incisions were made, one alongside and to the left of the sagittal sinus, and one behind the left hair line. They both yielded discoloured, brownish, purulent, exudate, with many pus cells and g + cocci under the microscope. The diagnosis was frontal subaponeurotic cellulitis. Search for syphilis was negative. There were no abnormal neurological findings. The patient was kept under hospital observation for 4 months during which period the process settled down spontaneously. No signs of intracranial spread developed. He was discharged without complaints and was left with small scars from the incisions mentioned. Radiologically, there was no progress in the involvement of the bone.

Case 1.19. POTT's puffy tumour of acute onset with high temperature, leading eventually to drowsiness, and clearing up spontaneously within 6 weeks. No clinical signs of paranasal sinus infection.

A girl of 12 years had complained, for about 8 days, of increasing frontal headaches and a tender swelling on her forehead; she did not vomit but gradually became drowsy. The admission diagnosis was: doubtful frontal sinusitis; (?) sagittal sinus thrombosis with frontal abscess. On examination, she was lethargic and had a stiff neck and a pyrexia up to 103° F. The scalp on her forehead was thickened and pitting from the coronal suture down including the upper and lower lids of both eyes and both zygomatic regions. The area of the glabella was fluctuant and tender on pressure; the tenderness extended over both supraorbital regions. There was no discharge from the nose or from the ears. Fundoscopy revealed a mild congestion of both papillae. No localising signs were present. On the X-ray plates of the skull the frontal sinus was very small on either side and it was suggested that what presented as such, were really enlarged ethmoid cells. The structure of the frontal bone was intact.

A small incision above the nose revealed a normal bone and beneath the periosteum some purulent debris. A small area of dura mater was exposed and found normal. Another incision was made into the fluctuating area over the glabella with similar findings. The patient was discharged with linear scars and without complaints, at the end of a 6 weeks' stay at the hospital.

Concluding remarks on frontal osteitis, Pott's "Puffy Tumour", and subdural empyema in frontal region

a) Age incidence

From Table 1 it will be seen that the younger age group is predominantly involved. 7 out of 8 cases were under 15 years af age and, if the two cases of rhinogenic frontal abscess (cases 1.5 and 1.2) are included, it follows that 9 out of the 10 cases were under the age of 20.

b) Pathogenesis

Relation to frontal sinus infection is rather obvious and confirms earlier findings with regard to frontal subdural abscess (COURVILLE, 1950; BOTTERELL and DRAKE, 1952; WEBER, 1957). In the present series frontogenic etiology was suggested in 5 out of the 10 cases by opacity of the frontal sinus (or its equivalents) on the X-rays, and previous history.

Frontogenic origin of the infection may be somewhat obscured in infants and children by the absence of a proper frontal sinus in this age group. In the above series the frontal sinus was found twice replaced, on exposure, by what appeared to be an enlarged ethmoid cell adjoining the medial part of the orbit (cases 1.17 and 1.19). In the majority of cases presented here, the history and findings suggested an acute and even fulminating infection of the accessory air sinuses thus confirming COURVILLE's conclusions drawn from a series of 42 cases of frontogenic subdural empyema (1944). Exacerbation of a chronic sinus infection, as emphasized by KUBIK and ADAMS, was suggested but not established beyond doubt in case 1.18.

c) Differential diagnosis

A tentative diagnosis of intraorbital phlegmon, oedema or abscess is made, not infrequently, in these patients when handed over first to the eye specialist or the otologist. Diagnosis of acute cavernous sinus thrombosis may be suggested by acute onset and local signs, and, in fact, was a complicating factor in two patients of the present series (cases 1.20 and 1.21) as indicated by definite neurological findings.

Tuberculous meningitis was suspected in one case (case 1.23) but soon disproved by the absence of relevant signs in the lumbar fluid.

In cases with insidious onset and protracted course revealing, on the X-ray films, a "mottled" appearance of the frontal squama due to patchy sclerosis and rarefication of bone, such as in cases 1.18 and 1.16, serological tests for syphilis may be indicated; in the older age group secondaries of the skull should be considered a possibility.

Epileptic seizures frequently occur in subdural abscess. They were present in 14 of the 42 cases in COURVILLE's series (1944). ERASMUS has emphasized their importance in differential diagnosis from brain abscess. Also WEBER (1950) in his series of six subdural abscesses has found unilateral jacksonian fits in four. In two of the three patients with subdural empyema included in the present series epileptic discharges of the jacksonian or the continuous type were observed and judged indicative of the lesion (cases 1.17 and 1.23); in both the clinical course was fulminating and the convulsions, difficult to bring under control, imperceptibly merged into a preterminal status epilepticus. No seizures of any kind were noticed in the infant (case 1.22) with the post-meningitic subdural abscess.

d) Intracranial complications

The three patients with subdural empyema have just been mentioned. Thrombosis of the superior sagittal sinus and the superior cerebral veins have been found, at autopsy, to be a rather common complication indicating the path of extension in subdural empyema (COURVILLE, 1944 and 1950). COURVILLE also illustrated such venous thrombosis opening up a two-way avenue into the subdural as well as the subarachnoid spaces.

In case 1.17 of our series a recent thrombosis of the superior sagittal sinus extending into the right lateral and sigmoid sinuses was found on the post mortem table and, under the microscope, scattered intramural abscesses were disclosed in addition. It may be suggested that, in this case, formation of cortical abscesses was precluded by the fulminating course.

Thrombosis of the major dural sinuses as in case 1.17 has a significant analogue in penetrating wounds of the fronto-basal area, and we shall return to this point in discussing case 1.7 in the section on war injuries.

The two frontogenic brain abscesses in which signs of frontal osteitis preceded intracranial suppuration have been discussed under Group I (cases 1.5 and 1.2). They may be pictured as two prototypes of pathogenesis and clinical development of frontogenic cerebral abscess representing, the one (case 1.5), a continuous course and contiguous spread of infection to reach, finally, the brain substance; the other (case 1.2), exemplifying a larval stage of frontal epicranial infection resulting in dependent oedema and peri-orbital abscess formation, and followed, after a significant time lapse, by signs of an intracranial mass.

e) Outcome

Mild cases such as instanced by the case histories 1.16 and 1.19 with the infection restricted to the frontal bone and the epicranium, present no surgical problem. Of those with intracranial complications five patients died, viz. the two frontal abscesses, and three cases complicated by acute subdural empyema. Regarding the latter, the small series of the present record compares unfavourably, it must be admitted, with larger series reported by others. Thus, GURDJIAN and WEBSTER (1948b) had no fatality in four cases. BOTTERELL and DRAKE (1952) treated successfully ten patients four of whom had associated brain abscess. WEBER's series (1957) includes 12 patients with acute subdural empyema; the first five died but were followed by seven survivals.

In our three patients multiple trephine openings were made and penicillin instilled intradurally in an attempt to remove the pent-up pus and to sterilize the subdural space. These attempts failed probably because of complicating lesions, such as dural sinus thrombosis and septic meningitis. It is significant that two patients died in status epilepticus and with signs of septicaemia not responding to antibiotics in common use at the time (1955 and 1956). It has been proved, however, in the one case (1.17) by necropsy that complete removal of a subdural abscess including its pyogenic membrane is possible and, in fact, had been achieved on the one side. It is obvious that this is practicable only provided the pus is not too thick to be removed by suction, and in the absence of fibrinous adhesions between the dura mater and the pia-arachnoid resulting in multiple abscesses and at sites difficult to approach surgically. In case 1.22 the drainage probably was inadequate and resulted in brain stem shift with increasing obstruction of the cerebrospinal fluid passages.

II. The fronto-basal injuries. Groups III and IV

The foremost surgical problem here is dural involvement, its diagnosis, implications and operative repair. The dura mater has been recognized as the essential protective barrier against bacterial invasion of the brain and meninges long before the First World War, and this resulted, during the war, in the principle of excision and primary closure of head wounds as elaborated by CUSHING, BARANY, GULEKE and others[1].

Primary suture of battle wounds, however, has met with serious drawbacks and has by no means been generally accepted; under the conditions of war, it proved impracticable to carry it out within the required time-limit of twelve hours, and with a surgical staff often limited to the utmost; too rapidly, the period of bacterial contamination of the wound changed into one of bacterial tissue invasion (JEFFERSON, 1947). So, the "open" treatment of penetrating head wounds, with or without drainage, remained an alternative widely practised, and involving, almost invariably, cerebral fungus formation with its inherent sequelae i.e. additional damage to the brain and intra-dural infection.

The position was somewhat different with regard to injuries involving the paranasal sinuses, Here, from experiences in civilian neurosurgery, dural involvement has been emphasized as the essential factor in prognosis and treatment before and at the very beginning of the Second World War (CAIRNS, 1937 and 1942; TÖNNIS and his team, 1941; SORGO, 1942; CALVERT, 1942), and on either side of the war frontiers. So, early dural repair became an accepted principle in this type of injury, and, together with the newly acquired resources of chemotherapy, resulted in a drop of incidence of severe intracranial infections undreamed of before (see section on "War Injuries").

1. Criteria of dural involvement in fronto-basal injury

Generally speaking clinical observation proves to be a more reliable guide as to the penetrating nature of the wound than intricate X-ray diagnostic manoeuvres valuable though these may be.

---

[1] CUSHING's paper appeared in Brit. J. Surg. 5, 558 (1918). An excellent survey on war injuries is given by G. JEFFERSON in: Head Wounds and Infection in Two Wars; Brit. J. Surg. War Surgery. Suppl. No. 1. Wounds of the Head (1947), p. 3 et seq.
R. BARANY: Brun's Beitr. klin. Chir. 97, 397 (1915). N. GULEKE: Münch. med. Wschr. 29, 989 (1915); Ergebn. Chir. Orthop. 10, 116/195 (1918). The German surgeons summarized their experiences on brain injuries during the First World War in: O. v. SCHERNING's Handbuch der ärztlichen Erfahrungen im Weltkriege. Band VIII. Leipzig: J. A. Barth 1922.

Anosmia, or some degree of it, has been emphasized long ago by SPATZ, in studying local cortical contusions at definite sites of predilection, as an important neurological finding, too often neglected in head injuries in civil life. It was re-emphasized by TÖNNIS (1941) and CALVERT (1942) with regard to war injuries. Unfortunately, testing of smell sensation often fails in unintelligent and inco-operative patients, and those with impaired consciousness.

Anosmia, one-sided or complete, together with other signs suggesting damage to the bony walls of the accessory sinuses, were considered a definite indication for operation by most neurosurgeons at the beginning of the last war (JOHNSON and DUTT). Such bony involvement is evinced by visible bone splinters or disrupted skull fragments in an open wound over the sinuses, by pulsation or bulge of the adjacent parts, and especially by surgical emphysema with its crepitus on palpation, most conspicuous over the loose fronto-orbital tissues.

Linear fractures and isolated fissures involving the orbital roof extension of the frontal sinus must be born in mind, especially in blunt injuries and at a distance from the point of force inflicted, as demonstrated experimentally by GURDJIAN and LISSNER in 1944, and clearly confirmed later on the X-ray plates by JOHNSON and DUTT, 1947, and on the post mortem table by KLAUE, 1948. Thus, among 22 meningeal haemorrhages of traumatic origin reported on by the author (IRSIGLER, 1957), there were three cases of unsuspected fissuring of the floor of the anterior and middle fossae disclosed at necropsy: all three had fractures of both orbital roofs, associated, in two, with a fissure through the right petrous bone, and, in one, with a shattered ethmoid. No meningitis was present in these cases.

Cerebro-spinal leak, either profuse or as a scanty, watery or blood-stained discharge, may occur from the open wound, through the nostrils, into the nasopharynx, or — rarely — into the orbital tissues. SCHLOFFER was the first to describe traumatic otorrhoea. It may be evident only in the upright or face-down position of the patient. Not infrequently, it is initiated by blowing the nose or sneezing. There may be a broad communication into the nasopharynx without the injured being aware of any watery discharge there, even if he is fully conscious and co-operative; posterior rhinoscopy is needed to disclose it (case 1.13).

Brain tissue may extrude from the wound or into a crevice beneath a raised part of the scalp or a dislodged flake of bone, plugging a dural tear and visible only on debridement of the wound. In gunshot injuries pieces of brain tissue may be found in the upper pharynx or on expectoration.

In intra-cranial aeroceles of some size and filled in part with cerebro-spinal fluid a tympanitic area on percussion of the overlying vault, and a conspicuous splashing noise on shaking the patient's head may be diagnostic (case 1.8). Both signs were mentioned by KASPAR[1] as early as 1936. An intra-cranial air cyst or a pneumocephaly of traumatic origin may be easily missed on the X-ray plates if not carefully looked for; in one of the author's patients the diagnosis was made from a tiny air bubble within the pontine cistern.

Finally, *X-ray examination* may be of great assistance in assessment of bony and dural involvement. If the patient's condition permits more elaborate projections to visualize the boundaries of the paranasal sinuses and the details of the floor of the anterior fossa, these will give valuable information. JOHNSON and DUTT, in a careful study (1947) emphasized oblique views of the ethmoids to demonstrate minute fissures and defects in this region.

KRÜGER (1959) has made X-ray findings a basic principle of classification and a rule-of-thumb guide to indications for surgery. It should be remembered however, that X-ray examination may not be contributory because the patient's condition does not permit time-consuming positioning to bring out intricate details such as tiny chips of bone so often responsible for dural tears (case 1.9). It is through such dural defects, difficult to find even on exposure, in association with dislodged bone splinters that infection gains access to the meninges; it is obvious that they may be responsible for operative failures.

---

[1] Quoted from VARA-LOPEZ, R., and J. SOLIS (1941), p. 49.

In one of the author's cases (case 1.17) who was admitted many months after a half-forgotten injury and with a history of bouts of meningitis, a tiny fracture of the posterior wall of the frontal sinus with displacement of a fragment into the latter gave, on the X-ray plates, the impression of an osteoma of the frontal sinus.

2. Implications of dural involvement

a) Early meningitis

It should be stressed from the outset that an open wound or a dural leakage are not a conditio sine qua non of an early meningitis developing within a fortnight from injury. There may be only a minor cut present or a bruise, in the orbito-facial region. Also X-ray films such as in common use, may be negative or non-contributory. However, it is general experience that the more extensive the damage to the bone as evinced by the X-rays the greater are the chances of an early meningitis.

The time factor, here, is of considerable importance.

CAIRNS, CALVERT, DANIEL, and NORTHCROFT, in their paper on infectious complications of head wounds (1947) have emphasized that swelling brain by plugging a dural tear commonly prevents infection from gaining access intradurally for the first few days; obviously, the same may be effected by dislodged bone or a foreign body or a clot, and in fact, in the majority of cases, meningitis develops after the fourth say, due to "unplugging" of the tear in the dura mater or from contaminated material displaced beneath the dura by the force afflicted during injury.

Clinical symptoms of meningitis may, however, develop as early as 48 hours following injury, and on the 3rd day a full-blown purulent meningitis, basal and over the convexity, has been found on the post mortem table, and also in cases without direct ventricular involvement which, according to CAIRNS and his coworkers, as a rule is responsible for the meningitis developing during the first three days. This applies equally to accident cases and to war injuries (TÖNNIS, 1941). See also Figs. 7 and 24.

Modern chemotherapy undoubtedly lowers the fatality rate and severity of intradural infection but, even with adequate dosage, does not eradicate it.

The points under discussion will be illustrated by the following case histories which will be given in some detail in view of the fact that it is the cases which, without having skin laceration, yet are compound into the nose or the accessory sinuses, have given rise to some controversy as to the necessity and time of surgical intervention.

Instances of early meningitis corroborating the point at issue are illustrated in Figs. 7 and 24.

Case 1.25. Meningitis with fatal outcome within 58 hours following injury to the forehead in a man who was admitted with a bruise over the left eye. No rhinorrhoea. Necropsy: Multiple fractures of the floor of the anterior fossa.

An African male was admitted with a small cut wound over the left eye; the upper lid of the eye was suffused, and there were bruises over the right shoulder and knee. He was unconscious and so restless as to require paraldehyde for sedation. His condition excluded X-ray examination. He was put on penicillin and sulphadiazine in adequate doses and died without regaining consciousness, 58 hours after admission.

On the post mortem table the following findings were made: fracture of the left orbital roof extending into the frontal sinus and involving the lamina cribriformis. Intraorbital haematoma on the left. Diffuse fibrino-purulent meningitis on the base as well as over the convexity, creamy yellowish pus distending the basal cisterns and the 4th ventricle. Pronounced cerebellar coning on both sides. — Small extradural clot on the floor of the left anterior fossa. Small cortical contusion over the left temporal pole and over the right occipital lobe. No petechiae on the cut surface through the brain stem.

Case 1.26. Purulent meningitis within two days in a man who had received a blow into his face with bruises and abrasions around his nose and eyes. No open wound. Initial and transient rhinorrhoea. Recovery after frontal craniotomy and dural repair.

A European man, aged 22, suffered an injury to his forehead and was knocked unconscious but regained consciousness after a short while. There was apparent fracture of his nose and both orbital regions were bruised. It was reported that some blood together with small air bubbles had been discharged from his nostrils after the blow. No open wound was present. Radiologically, the fracture extended into the floor of the anterior fossa. Exploratory burr holes performed in a country hospital in search for a clot were negative. Chemotherapy was instituted. Two days after the injury the lumbar fluid was found to contain pus; the patient improved gradually under intravenous achromycin, he became co-operative and well orientated, and his temperature dropped to normal although there was still neck rigidity. A conspicuous herpetic eruption appeared on the lips and the adjacent areas of the face, more so on the left. There was no discharge from the nose and the ears; the right nostril was blocked with scabs of encrusted blood. No localising signs were present on neurological examination.

Eight days after the injury an osteoplastic flap was turned down on the right. The dura mater was under marked tension. The right anterior horn was needled and emptied, it contained clear fluid. The cribriform plate was approached extradurally and found shattered on either side of the crista galli part of which had broken loose but was left in situ. Minute bony splinters were dislodged and had pierced through the dura mater; cerebrospinal fluid was leaking through several small openings. The cribriform area was exposed in its entire extent by stripping the dura off the floor of the anterior fossa. Two free grafts from the temporalis fascia were then tucked in loosely between dura and bone; no stitches were used to keep the grafts in situ. The posterior wall of the frontal sinus was intact. The dura mater was not incised and was pulsating nicely. The bone flap was resutured to the periosteum and the wound closed in the usual way. No antibiotics were used topically. Wound healing was per primary union. As far as it is known the patient remained well since 1958.

b) Intracranial hypotension

Intracranial low pressure state, also referred to as "aliquorrhoea" (SCHALTENBRAND) is an accepted though not common sequel to trauma to the head. If not related to some sort of cerebro-spinal leak its etiology is open to some speculation. Occasionally, it may follow a pre-existing dehydration due to excessive fluid loss, to lumbar puncture, or ventricular tap. It is a definite factor in the formation of subdural collections, especially clots of traumatic origin and following craniotomies. It is also related as one would expect to ventricular collapse; but, here, it is doubtful whether the relation is that of cause or effect.

ALLEN has postulated a kind of reflex "feedback" to the effect that production of cerebro-spinal fluid is controlled in some way by the hydrostatic pressure within the ventricles at any given time; consequently, if the intraventricular pressure drops below a certain level causing the ventricles to collapse fluid production would cease. This interesting speculation as yet lacks quantitative and experimental proof.

It is not clear whether, as suggested by SPROCKHOFF[1], some kind of damage to the choroid plexus accounts for intracranial hypotension following head trauma. However this may be a slack dura found on debridement of a penetrating head injury or in the course of evacuation of a posttraumatic intracranial clot always must arouse suspicion of a concealed cerebro-spinal leak. Such state of affairs has important diagnostic as well as therapeutic consequences apart from the obvious implication of a possible dural involvement with all its consequences regarding intradural spread of infection. Fortunately, it may considerably facilitate surgical approach and operative repair of a torn dura as SCHORSTEIN (1947) in discussing intracerebral haematoma in missile wounds has expressed it: "the lowering of pressure may convert a most difficult technical problem into a relatively simple one".

The suggestion by TÖNNIS to make use of repeated lumbar punctures for reposition of a cerebral fungus at certain stages of its development has been followed and confirmed by many others (see cases 1.3 and 1.7 in "War Injuries").

CONNOLLY (1956), in reporting on 4 cases of his own has pointed out that intracranial hypotension is likely to obscure the clinical picture following head trauma by preventing signs of raised pressure from becoming manifest, as well as the surgeon from being on his look-out for an extradural or subdural clot to be evacuated in time. The following three case histories already briefly referred to by the author in his paper on extradural haemorrhages in 1958, will serve to illustrate the points raised above and add somewhat to the picture by showing conclusively that acute intracranial hypotension associated with blunt injury to the head may easily pave the way for fatal extradural and/or subdural haematomas.

Case 1.31. Death occurred within a couple of hours in a man who had suffered a heavy blow to his forehead resulting in multiple fractures of the frontal bone and sinus. No overt rhinorrhoea. The man was unconscious

---

[1] H. SPROCKHOFF's papers were not available to me at present. They appeared in Nervenarzt 13, 341 (1940), and in Arch. klin. Chir. 200, 185 (1940).

throughout with signs of brain stem damage from the onset. Extradural and subdural haematomas at the site of contrecoup.

An African male, aged 36, was admitted deeply unconscious and in poor condition after having suffered a heavy blow against his forehead. There was a small cut, hardly one inch long, above his left eye brow surrounded by an area of crepitus on palpation indicating surgical emphysema which extended into the left upper eye lid. Also the lower lid of this eye was bruised and suffused. There was blood oozing from his nostrils and his mouth. The pupils were maximally dilated and fixed. Breathing was noisy and strenuous. The patient did not react to painful stimuli, his limbs were slack, the reflexes, including abdominals and plantars, were absent. Skull X-rays revealed a stellate and depressed fracture of the frontal bone on the left involving the frontal sinus which, in this patient, was particularly large. He died two hours after admission. *Autopsy* disclosed a comminuted fracture of the floor of the anterior fossa extending upward into the calvaria. The significant finding was a contrecoup contusion of the right occipital lobe together with an extradural as well as a subdural clot of considerable extent at the same site. No pressure cone and no pontine haemorrhages were present to the naked eye.

Comment. A fulminating extradural and subdural haematoma had developed in this case, and resulted, together with the damage to the brain stem (as indicated neurologically), in the patient's death within two hours of admission. It would appear that immediate and profuse cerebrospinal fluid leak occurred through the shattered floor of the anterior fossa followed by intracranial hypotension which, in its turn, facilitated formation of the two clots. It is to be noted that the double haemorrhage was in close relation to a contrecoup lesion of the occipital lobe of the brain. No fracture was present at that site.

Case 1.32. Compound fracture of the anterior fossa with disruption of the frontal sinus. No overt rhinorrhoea. Operation on admission with the patient fully conscious under local anaesthesia. Dura mater slack. Debridement and primary closure. One hour later sudden death in status epilepticus. Necropsy: Contrecoup subdural haemorrhage over the occipital lobes. No signs of coning on the post mortem table.

A 32-year-old African male was hit several times with an ax on his left forehead when engaged in a brawl, he was reported to have stumbled to the ground but had not been knocked out. When admitted to the ward on the following day i.e. 18 hours after the incident he was responsive and able to relate details of what had happened. There was a broad cut wound, $2^1/_2$ in. in length, extending obliquely over the left frontal area and surrounded by some minor cuts. The left eye was heavily bruised and with a conjunctival haemorrhage in the lateral angle. The upward movements of this eye were somewhat restricted. Both pupils were middle-sized, equal, and reacting to light. There were no neurological deviations, nor was there any discharge from the nose. X-rays of the skull revealed a comminuted fracture of the left frontal bone extending both into the frontal sinus and into the base of the skull. The frontal sinus was opaque throughout, with indistinct boundaries. Numerous scattered air bubbles were visible over the convexity and within the basal cisterns, on either side of the falx cerebri; also the left frontal horn contained a tiny bit of air (Fig. 17).

Operation was performed on admission under local anaesthesia. The big cut on the left side of the forehead was enlarged so as to encompass the right frontal region. When a wound retractor was inserted air bubbles escaped from the depth of the wound. The left half of the frontal sinus was disrupted and wide open, loose bone pieces were extracted from within the sinus. The left orbital roof was shattered too but was left in situ. Both the outer and the inner table of the cranial vault were broken down and depressed into the anterior and the middle fossae. The exposed dura was slack; on stripping it off the floor, no tear could be demonstrated. There was no fracture of the ethmoid bone to the naked eye. What was left of the bony walls of the frontal sinus was duly rounded off with a rongeur and the lining mucosal membrane removed with a curette. The intact dura mater was then covered with gelatin foam. After sprinkling the wound with penicillin powder two soft rubber drains were issued through button holes on either side of the main incision. Then the wound was closed in two layers. During the whole procedure the patient was conscious and responsive. He started complaining of pain and became rather restless during cleansing out the frontal sinus and, at this stage, required a small amount of pentothal sodium to supplement local anaesthesia. When leaving the operation table his condition was quite satisfactory. One hour later he developed right-sided jacksonian fits which rapidly became generalised and ended in respiratory failure.

Post mortem examination revealed a cerebral contusion over the right occipital area underlying an extensive subdural haematoma which covered both occipital lobes. There were no signs of tentorial or cerebellar pressure cone and, to the naked eye, no haemorrhages within the brain stem were present.

Comment. Here again, as in the foregoing case an unsuspected contusion of the brain at the site of contrecoup was associated with an acute, and fatal subdural haematoma extending, in this case, over both occipital lobes. Though no rhinorrhoea was present and no dural tear found on exposure, a concealed cerebrospinal fluid leak, possibly through the lacerated wound on the forehead over the frontal sinus, is evinced by the slackness of the dura mater as found during debridement. Death from respiratory failure occurred in status epilepticus ushered in by jacksonian fits in the fully conscious patient, one hour after completion of the operation.

The absence of pressure cone and of mesencephalic haemorrhages in this and the foregoing case seems to indicate that it is the acute interference with cortical function rather than with the vital centres in the brain stem which is responsible for the fatal outcome. This obviously does not mean that absence of gross lesions in the brain stem will rule out any damage at a neuronal level at this site. JEFFERSON, in discussing "The Balance of Life and Death in Cerebral Lesions" (1957) reports on a 12-year-old boy who had two cerebellar tuberculomas and died in coma 5 days after posterior fossa exploration. He had clear signs of serious brain stem damage as well as what the author calls "low level convulsions" indicating local excitation of the reticular area. On the post mortem table no haemorrhages were present anywhere in the midbrain, pons, or medulla but imminent constriction at this crucial point of the neuraxis was indicated by the presence of an upward tentorial herniation of unusual size.

Case 1.36. Fronto-basal injury with small laceration above left eye. No dural leak. Blood in lumbar fluid. KOJEWNIKOW's continuous epilepsy from the 4th day on resulting, within 24 hours, in hyperpyrexia and death. Necropsy: Subdural haematoma in posterior fossa. Laceration of both frontal lobes. Subarachnoid and intraventricular bleeds. Fresh blood in trachea.

An adult African male was admitted in a state of restless stupor and without a history being available. There was a small scalp laceration above the left eye-brow which had been stitched up superficially. The pupils

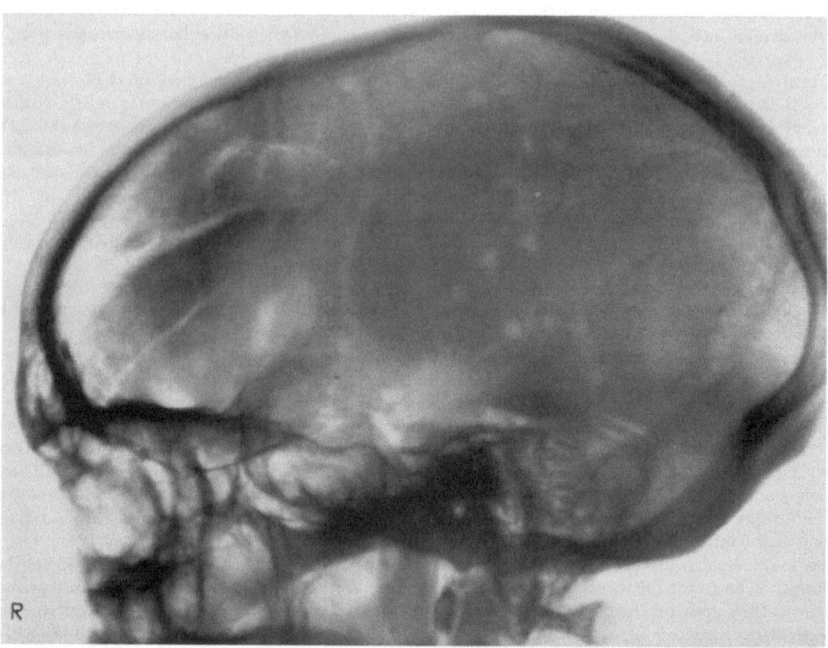

Fig. 17. Compound fracture of the forehead involving the frontal sinus and base of skull alike. Note air within the basal cisterns and left anterior horn exemplifying traumatic air encephalogram. (Case 1.32)

were equal, the neck stiff, and the left arm and leg were hemiplegic. The patient was able to swallow; he was incontinent. Roentgen photos of the skull exhibited a depressed fracture of the left frontal bone involving the frontal sinus; the latter was densely shadowed. No external cerebrospinal fluid leak could be detected. Chemotherapy was installed. Lumbar taps yielded pure blood at first; later the fluid became less blood-stained but with an increasing number of polymorphs. No organisms were found in the lumbar fluid and the culture remained sterile. On the 4th day following admission the patient developed almost continuous left-sided convulsions of the characteristic KOJEWNIKOW's type, involving his face, arm, and hand but not his leg and requiring high doses of barbiturates. The lumbar fluid now became again heavily blood-stained, the coma deepened and there was profuse sweating; the temperature gradually climbed to high levels. The patient died within 24 hours after the onset of convulsions, 5 days after admission.

The following were the findings on the post mortem table: Comminuted fracture of the left frontal bone with contusions and lacerations of both frontal lobes, more so on the left, and minor contusions of the temporal poles. There was a wide-spread subarachnoid bleed with blood within the 4th ventricle. Finally, an extensive subdural haematoma was found occupying the posterior fossa. No meningitis was noticed. There was fresh blood in the trachea.

Comment. There can be little doubt that in this case, which was complicated by a subarachnoid haemorrhage, the formation of so rare a condition as a subdural clot within the posterior fossa was facilitated by a concealed cerebrospinal fluid leak probably into the pharynx as indicated by the presence of blood within the trachea at necropsy five days after the injury. Obviously, such a leak is easily overlooked in a patient in persistent stupor and being nursed while lying face upward. Detailed radiological examination to show the extent of the fronto-basal fracture was not practicable because of the patient's poor condition throughout. It is also worth mentioning that after 5 days and despite a shattered frontal sinus no frank meningitis was found on post mortem examination and the lumbar fluid remained sterile up to the end; surely, chemotherapy here played its part.

The Lesson emerging from the foregoing case histories seems to be that in patients with fronto-basal injury and extensive fracture of the floor of the anterior fossa, even in the absence of an open wound and an overt dural leak, one has to be constantly on the watch for an acute contre-coup clot, outside and/or below the dura mater, which most likely will be found in the occipital region or even within the posterior fossa. Convulsions, at first jacksonian and later becoming generalised or of the continuous (KOJEWNIKOW's) type to end in status epilepticus, are almost diagnostic of such dural haemorrhage and should, at any rate, induce urgent explorative burr holes. Owing to the low pressure state prevailing in these patients even a small clot may rapidly grow to a magnitude interfering with either the function of the cerebral cortex as heralded by the transition into status epilepticus, or alternately, with function of the vital centres in the brain stem.

Table 2. *Synopsis of 10 cases in group III*

Case no.	Diagnosis of frontobasal injury established	Operation	Course
1.25	Autopsy: fracture of left orbital roof extending into frontal sinus and cribriform plate	No	Died within 58 hours; diffuse fibrinopurulent meningitis
1.27	X-rays: linear fracture through right frontal bone Autopsy: depressed fronto-orbital fracture extending into ethmoid	Superficial sutures, no dural repair	Died 6 days after injury in status epilepticus; pus in basal cisterns and ventricles
1.28	X-rays: depressed fracture left frontal with frontal sinus involved	Operation on admission; two tears in dura; dura slack; dural repair, primary closure	Recovered; wound healed per primary union
1.31	Surgical emphysema around left eye	No	Died within 2 hours from contre-coup extradural and subdural clots
1.32	Spontaneous pneumencephalo-gram	Debridement on admission including frontal sinus	Died one hour following operation in status epilepticus from contre-coup subdural haemorrhage
1.34	Fronto-basal depressed fracture extending into frontal sinus and ethmoid	Debridement on admission; dura slack (intact ?)	Recovered with primary wound healing
1.36	Fronto-basal depressed fracture on left; wound above left eye brow sutured	No	Purulent meningitis within 3 days; convulsions and left hemiplegia; died after 5 days from subdural haemorrhage in posterior fossa and contusion of frontal lobes
1.37	Depressed and comminuted left fronto-basal fracture incl. ethmoid; anterior fossa shattered	Dural repair day after admission; contusion of left frontal lobe	Primary wound healing; recovered
1.38	Surgical emphysema of left upper eye lid; no X-rays done; initial rhinorrhoea subsided spontaneously	Operation about 11 months after injury; left fronto-temporal flap; subdural aerocele filled with CSF. and air; gliosed brain (biopsy)	Recovered
1.40	Depressed fronto-basal fracture adjacent to frontal sinus	Operation on 3rd day; dura torn; exenteration of frontal sinus; dural repair	Recovered with primary wound healing

3. Group III: Fronto-basal fracture with dural involvement but without "overt" cerebrospinal fluid leak

In Table 2 the individual features of the 10 cases in this group are summarized. Half of the patients have succumbed soon or within 6 days following admission.

Comment. (a) With regard to the survivals the following points emerge:

1. All patients who were operated on survived with one exception (case 1.32) who died from a contre-coup subdural clot shortly after operation that was performed on admission.

2. Three of the five cases who recovered were operated upon on admission or within 24 hours following admission. One (case 1.40) underwent operation on the 3rd day; one (case 1.38) who had no open wound but a surgical emphysema which was aspirated after injury was operated upon 11 months later.

The scalp lacerations of these patients though in part badly contused and contaminated, healed without exception per primary union after surgical debridement under chemotherapeutic "cover". This confirms earlier experiences by SCHORSTEIN (1944) in compound fronto-orbital fractures.

b) Regarding the fatalities the following points are noteworthy:

1. Among the five fatalities there were 4 who had no operation performed.

2. There were 2 early fatalities (cases 1.32 and 1.31) dying within a few hours after admission, both from contre-coup subdural haemorrhage; one of them (case 1.32) who had a spontaneous pneumencephalogram succumbed one hour after debridement of his wound.

3. The 3 late fatalities (cases 1.25, 1.27, and 1.36) who succumbed on the 3rd day after admission or later had purulent meningitis which was the cause of death in two; one patient (case 1.36) with contusion of both frontal lobes died on the 5th day from a sub-dural haemorrhage in the posterior fossa in addition to his meningitis.

The *Conclusions* arrived at from the foregoing cases of group III appear then to be the following:

a) Early and final surgical approach is indicated in all cases with fronto-basal fractures involving the air sinuses or with signs of dural involvement such as intracranial air collections or surgical emphysema in the fronto-orbital region irrespective of the presence or absence of an open wound or frank cerebrospinal fluid leakage.

b) The possibility of an acute intracranial haemorrhage, extradural or subdural, should constantly be born in mind and adequate measures taken in time, exploratory burrholes being indicated at the site of contre-coup i.e. over the occipital lobes and the posterior fossa.

4. Group IV: Fronto-basal fracture with cerebrospinal fluid leak

There are 12 cases and no death in this Group. In Table 3 the main points of each case history are outlined. They can be summarized as follows:

a) Early operation (à chaud)

Early operation within a fortnight after injury has been performed in 6 cases. All stood the procedure well, including

1. two cases (cases 1.4 and 1.26) who were operated upon on the 2nd and 8th days respectively, with manifest signs of meningitis (associated with herpes labialis) and evidenced by pus in, or positive culture from, lumbar fluid;

2. one (case 1.13) with naso-pharyngeal leak and a low grade meningitis, who was operated upon on the 9th day after injury;

3. one patient (case 1.29), also with a nasopharyngeal leak, who was operated upon 15 days after injury.

One patient (case 1.4), following initial delay of surgery, had a bout of meningitis and developed a left frontal abscess not associated with meningitis. His case history will be presented on p. 45 et seq.

Despite early operation, some degree of mental derangement is likely to develop.

b) Operation à froid

Craniotomy has been performed 4 weeks and more after the injury in 6 patients all of whom recovered; however, there was one immediate failure (case 1.10, p. 47) in whom the dural leak recurred following re-operation. He had evidence of severe brain damage and extensive ventricular dilatation. It is likely that follow-up studies carried out over a longer period than was possible in the present series would show a higher incidence of recurrences.

In one patient (case 1.11) the final outcome is unknown.

In one patient (case 1.14), aged 37, signs of cardiac infarction developed from which he recovered soon; however, progressive mental derangement within a few months following operation raised the question of sending him into a mental institution.

Table 3. *Synopsis of 12 cases in group IV*

Case no.	Diagnosis of frontobasal injury established	Operation	Course
1.4	Lacerated wound over forehead and comminuted fracture of frontal and ethmoid sinuses. Superficial sutures. Pneumococcal meningitis within two days	2 days after injury; dura pierced by fragment from ethmoid, stitched and sealed off with gelatine foam	Rapid recovery from meningitis; primary wound healing (Fig. 24). Frontal lobe syndrome. Died 21 months later from left frontal abscess without meningitis
1.8	Watery discharge from left nostril 2 or 3 days after injury	Laceration over left eye stitched; 6 weeks later signs of intracranial aerocele	Smooth Left frontal flap 9 weeks after injury, dural repair (Fig.25)
1.9	Rhinorrhoea on right and recurrent intracerebral aerocele	Dural repair; bone chips dislodged into brain	Cured
1.10	Recurrent rhinorrhoea on right; bilateral frontal aerocele and spontaneous pneumencephalogram; bilateral ventricular dilatation (cerebral atrophy); first fascial graft, 5 months previously, had failed	Re-exploration by right frontal flap; no dural defect found;? communication to sphenoid sinus	Failed again
1.11	Chronic recurrent intracerebral aerocele blowing up on sneezing etc.	Dural repair	Unknown
1.12	Chronic recurrent rhinorrhoea and meningitis; fracture of frontal sinus	Dural repair about one year after injury; brain herniating into frontal sinus	Recovered
1.13	Comminuted fracture of frontal and ethmoid sinuses; brain extruding; nasopharyngeal leak, low grade meningitis; fracture of right petrous bone	Dural repair on 9th day after injury	Recovered, healing per primary; slight psych-organic syndrome; anosmia; right deafness
1.14	Extensive laceration over forehead, depressed fracture extending into frontal and ethmoid sinuses. Poor condition on admission; superficial sutures. 3 weeks later rhinorrhoea and spontaneous pneumencephalogram.	Right frontal flap 4 weeks after injury; intracerebral aerocele and contusion of frontal lobe; brain herniated and trapped within fragments. Dural closure	Attack of myocardial infarction; wound healing practically p.pr. intention. Severe psych-organic mentality 3 months later
1.26	No open wound, fronto-orbital bruises; fracture of nose and floor of anterior fossa; bloodstained rhinorrhoea; exploratory burr holes: no clot. Within 2 days lumbar tap purulent	Right frontal flap and dural repair on 8th day after injury, bone splinters piercing through dura	Recovered, wound healed practically p.pr.
1.29	No skin laceration, left blindness. Comminuted fracture of nose, left orbit, and floor of anterior fossa. Nasopharyngeal leak and scattered air bubbles in subarachnoid spaces	Dural repair 15 days after injury; bone splinters dislodged intradurally, brain damaged	Recovered
1.33	2 lacerations above eye brows stitched up superficially; depressed fracture of anterior and posterior walls of frontal sinus. CSF. leak from wound	Dura sutured and patched with orbital tissue	Per primary healing
1.35	Laceration over glabella; brain extruding; depressed fracture of frontal sinus	Operation 2 days after injury, numerous in-driven bone spiculae, dural tear adjacent to splintered crista galli; dural repair	CSF. oozing through drain on 2nd day; wound healed p.pr. 5 weeks later re-admitted with wound slightly gaping and fluctuating. Lumbar tap purulent. Recovered under antibiotics

In the majority of cases presented here, there is too little known about the pre-morbid personality, and the postoperative follow-up period is too short for final assessment of incidence and degree of behavioural disorders which developed after craniotomy. However, a permanent and even progressive mental derangement is not too a remote possibility, even after successful primary surgery (see case 1.4, p. 45).

Conclusions. 1. In all cases with manifest dural leak early operation within a fortnight following injury is indicated.

2. In patients undergoing re-exploration for a recurrent cerebrospinal fistula, often associated with intracranial air cysts and previous meningitic episodes, extensive frontal lobe damage must be taken into account as evidenced by ventricular dilatation. In cases not presenting with a spontaneous pneumencephalogram the degree of brain atrophy already present should be assessed beforehand by air studies.

5. The place of chemotherapy in penetrating fronto-basal injuries

1. Full-range chemotherapy right from the beginning as a preventive measure is imperative and irrespective of the presence of an open wound or cerebrospinal fluid leak. This applies especially to cases with delayed surgery either because of the poor condition of the patient, or lack of appropriate surgical facilities, and when surgery is deferred because signs of bone damage are equivocal and those of dural involvement are considered of "minor degree" and transient.

2. Early chemotherapy is a deciding factor in primary intention healing of scalp wounds; this applies equally to accident wounds in civil life and to war injuries (SCHOR-STEIN, 1944). In this respect, modern chemotherapy has truly revolutionized our previous views on the time-limited FRIEDREICH excision of wounds.

3. Except for the reasons mentioned under 1. it appears unjustified to postpone surgery while being confident that chemotherapy will prevent infection from spreading intra-durally once and forever. During the initial stage of wound contamination and early bacterial tissue invasion (JEFFERSON, 1947), chemotherapy at its best will check wound infection and keep meningitis at a low grade thus extending the accepted time-limit of surgery beyond the 3rd day; however, no kind of chemotherapy will prevent late manifestations (see p. 45 et seq.) from developing unless thorough surgical repair and closure is undertaken as soon as condition and circumstances allow craniotomy. Furthermore, it should be realised that chemotherapy may change the character of inflammatory reaction and amount of pent-up pus to such a degree as to obscure the clinical picture and delay unduly surgical intervention. There are no means of keeping the accessory sinuses and the upper air passages reasonably and permanently sterile, nor can in-driven bone fragments or devitalized tissue plugging a dural tear be prevented from becoming a nidus of late intra-dural infection. Even with the most modern resources of chemotherapy at hands, the statement held by STEWART and BOTTERELL in their study on craniofacial-orbital wounds (1947) remains conclusive; it reads:

"In the majority of cases, with the pre- and post-operative use of penicillin and sulphon-amides, complications resulting from incomplete operation outweigh in significance the dangers of delaying surgical treatment for three days or perhaps longer."

6. Surgical management

a) Indications for surgery

In cases of large fronto-orbital laceration and damage to the bone necessitating per se debridement and surgical repair the direct route through the original wound is the method of choice. It implies enlarging of the bony defect to such extent as to give adequate access to the dura as well as the floor of the anterior fossa on either side of the crista galli.

Generally, this can be achieved by extending the incision on one or both sides to form a unilateral or bilateral hinged flap, or by a supra-orbital cross-bow incision just above the eye brows. The X-ray films showing site and extension of the bony damage provide a better guide than the expected cosmetic result after the wound healing; nevertheless, the scar should be showing as little as possible. Whenever feasible, the supra-ciliary arch and part of the anterior wall of the frontal sinus should be spared. The procedure will be illustrated when discussing case 1.13 below.

In the absence of a wound or when such wounds are of minor degree not requiring surgical excision, the indications for operation involving, in this case, a frontal osteoplastic flap, are to a certain amount subject to debate. Clearly, the question whether to operate or not depends in such cases on the damage to the bone walls of the paranasal sinuses as well as on the the possibility of dural involvement.

From the above discussion of Groups III and IV it seems obvious that early surgery is imperative in all cases where involvement of the dura mater is suspected. This requires a more detailed discussion.

First of all, early surgery is called for in patients presenting with definite signs of a dural tear such as outlined above, irrespective of any signs of local injury to the soft parts and/or the bone in the fronto-orbital region; here, a smouldering, pre-existent infection of the air sinuses or the oro-nasopharynx may be an aggravating factor. With regard to cerebrospinal fluid leak, an initial watery or blood-stained discharge subsiding, under adequate chemotherapy, after a few days should be differentiated from frank rhinorrhoea or pharyngorrhoea lasting for more than a few days or making a delayed appearance, viz. after one week or more following injury; the latter type requires surgical intervention as soon as the diagnosis is established and the patient's condition permits craniotomy. This view is shared by CAIRNS (1937, 1942), VOSS, MICHAELSSON[1] and others, and opposed by ADSON (1941) and ADSON and UIHLEIN (1949). TÖNNIS and FROWEIN advocate early active treatment concluding from their experience in 31 cases of traumatic cerebrospinal fistula and intracranial pneumatocele. SCHORSTEIN (in 1944) suggested early operation in blunt injuries associated with fronto-orbital fracture.

In determining the presence and site of a cerebrospinal fluid leak intrathecal instillation of a non-irritating dye such as indigo carmine by the lumbar or cisternal routes may be of assistance to visualize the path of leak as shown in the case 1.10 (p. 47) of the present series; this procedure, however, may be misleading as to the side of leakage (CAIRNS, 1937).

Secondly, fractures, either depressed or comminuted, require primary exposure, debridement and inspection of the walls of the frontal sinus and the dura mater, even in those cases, where, on the X-ray films, involvement of the air sinuses is not evidenced (case 1.40, p. 41). Simple linear fractures and fissures neighbouring the frontal sinus should be viewed with a watchful eye; in the author's opinion, no harm can be done by exposing the bone in order to determine clearly the condition of the sinus and of the adjacent dura mater. Finally, an early meningitis, clinical or as evidenced by pleocytosis in, or positive culture from, the lumbar fluid, associated with any kind of injury to the fronto-orbital area should be regarded an absolute indication for surgical attack and careful search for a dural tear as soon as the patient's condition tolerates operation.

The following two case histories will serve to bear out some of the relevant points in delayed surgery in such cases.

Case 1.13. Right fronto-basal injury communicating with the nasopharynx. Brain extruding. Superficial debridement and wound closure. Final wound excision and dural repair on the 9th day. Recovery.

A man of 20, while driving his car crashed into a moving train and suffered a deep laceration on his right forehead. He was taken to a hospital and immediately operated upon. The surgeon attending to him reported: "Beneath a triradiate wound above the right eye there was a comminuted fracture involving the frontal sinus and with brain extruding through the lacerated dura. Some bone fragments were removed and the wound closed. The patient was put on penicillin." Three days later he was transferred to the neurosurgical service for operation. He was co-operative and well orientated. He was unable to remember details of his accident but reported that blood had oozed from his right ear and from his nose. The scalp over the right eye was bulging and pulsating, indicating a large bony defect. A slight serous discharge from the wound had become frankly purulent and mixed with cerebrospinal fluid within the previous two days. Culture from the discharge

---

[1] Quoted from TÖNNIS and FROWEIN (1952), loc. cit.

from the wound yielded haemolytic staphylococci sensitive to streptomycin. Both eyes were suffused and there was chemosis of the right eye. There was a slight nuchal rigor and some restriction of the upward movements of the right eye. Crusts of dried blood were noted around the nostrils and within the right auditory meatus. There was no watery discharge from these places. There was anosmia. Hearing on the right side was considerably diminished. On the X-rays there was an irregular trephine opening in the right frontal squama. The right supra-ciliar arch was depressed and shattered. There was a fracture through the floor of the anterior fossa involving the frontal sinus and the ethmoid bone alike, the latter being displaced backwards. Extension of the fracture to the left side could be seen. The frontal as well as the ethmoid sinuses were opaque. Numerous

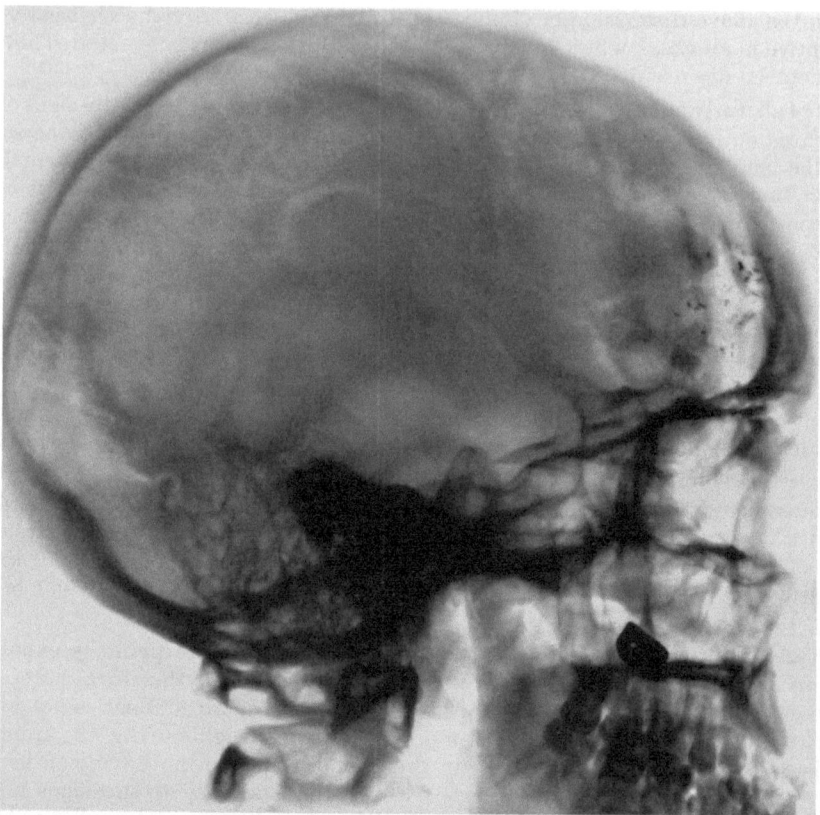

Fig. 18. Compound fracture through frontal sinus and floor of anterior fossa. Note in-driven bone fragments and metallic debris. Trephine opening in right frontal bone is due to the first, incomplete, surgical attempt. Final debridement and dural repair was carried out on the 9th day after injury (Case 1.13). See following Fig. 19

in-driven bone splinters and metallic debris were present in the injured area (Fig. 18). In addition, on the TOWNE's view, a fissure through the right petrous bone was visualised. The lumbar fluid was uniformly blood-stained, supernatent xanthochromic; pressure and dynamics were normal. Under the microscope some poly-morphonuclears and lymphocytes but no organisms were found; the culture was reported to be negative. Examination by the aural surgeon disclosed deafness on the right side. Posterior rhinoscopy revealed a broad communication with, and cerebrospinal fluid leak into, the right nasopharynx. While on the ward, the patient was on crystacillin and streptomycin 6 hourly.

Operative repair was undertaken on the 9th day after injury, under general anaesthesia. On re-opening the wound, a cup of necrotic brain tissue of pasty consistence was exposed and sucked off. Through a broad opening in the dura creamy brain tissue exuded. To get access to the brain, the trephine opening was enlarged so as to encompass the frontal sinus with its broken anterior and posterior walls. From it old clots and debris were cleansed out with the curette together with its mucosal lining. The right orbital roof was shattered. Four bone fragments of fair size were found dislodged on to the dura and beneath it within the brain itself. The healthy dura was exposed over the convexity and, as far as possible, on the floor of the anterior fossa but here, the dural defect extended too far backward to be brought into sight in its full extent. The dural edges were found firmly attached to the brain surface, thus shutting off the subdural and subarachnoid spaces from the infected area. No cerebrospinal fluid leak and no pus was found within the wound exposed. A free graft from the fascia lata was sutured onto the dura over the convexity and loosely tucked in, together with gelatine foam, between the brain and the bone to seal off the dural defect there. A free passage into the upper nasal meatus was then established and a brisk bleed from the ethmoidal arteries secured by compression with gelatine foam and thrombin. The fractured medial portion of the supra-ciliary arch was left in situ. Beneath the facial graft the brain pulsated nicely. The wound was sprinkled with penicillin powder and two rubber drains were issued through button holes on either side of the main wound which then was closed tightly in two layers.

All in all, this procedure took nearly 4 hours and was well stood by the patient. No blood transfusion was thought necessary. Streptomycin was continued.

The post-operative course was smooth, the wound healed practically per primary union and was pulsating over the bone defect. There was slight blood-stained discharge from the drains but no discharge from the nose. On the 4th post-operative day the lumbar fluid was clear and colourless, two lymphocytes and 30 mgm.% of protein were reported. The drains were removed on the 6th and 8th day respectively. Fig. 19 shows the patient on discharge from the hospital, 3 weeks after the operation. His only complaint then was headache on stooping. He was slightly euphoric and emotionally somewhat "flattened". There was complete anosmia and nearby deafness on the right side. Otherwise the neurological findings were within normal. One year after the operation a cranioplasty was performed with a satisfactory cosmetic result. He has remained well since (1955).

Comment. This patient, first of all, shows clearly the importance of chemotherapy when administered adequately and in time, in a case with incomplete primary debridement. The attending surgeon when seeing brain oozing throught a large dural defect into the fractured frontal sinus, was well-advised to close the wound after a superficial cleansing, and to refer the patient for final surgery to a neurosurgical ward. It is obvious that modern chemotherapy in such circumstances is a deciding factor in keeping the wound infection at a low grade; however, it does not prevent intradural spread of infection nor eliminate the danger of meningitis; therefore, it does not allow for "slackening down" the thoroughness of surgical repair.

Operation in this case exhibited also some of the difficulties to be faced, now and then, on delayed surgery. Spreading brain oedema due to extensive tissue damage, may prevent intracranial hypotension from developing in spite of a pharyngeal leak, and, moreover, may result in brain herniation and loss of a considerable part of the frontal lobe on one or even both sides. In extensive shattering of the anterior fossa the dural defect on the base may be so large as to preclude it from being viewed properly and repaired by painstaking sutures. It appears then preferable not to disrupt the adhesions between the dura and the brain already formed and to trust that a loose fascial graft put in between the brain and the bone, will prevent permanently communication with the air sinuses. The sealing

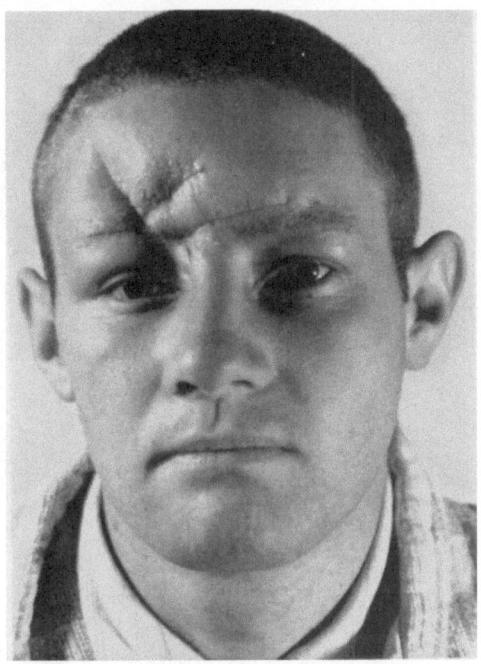

Fig. 19. This man crashed with his car into a moving train and suffered a deep laceration over the right forehead. The floor of the anterior fossa was shattered, brain tissue herniating through a hole in the dura, and CSF. oozing into the nasopharynx. Debridement and dural repair was carried out on the 9th day following the accident. Photo shows scar at the time of discharge from hospital. The cosmetic result was much improved by cranioplasty one year thereafter. Residual symptoms: slight frontal lobe euphoria and deafness on the right due to fracture of the petrous bone (Case 1.13)

off may be secured with gelatine foam or muscle as suggested by KRÜGER (1943). He issued a rubber drain through the nostrils if debridement of a shattered ethmoid bone resulted per se in a free passage into the nose. In the light of later experience and with the aid of more potent chemotherapeutic agents, it would now seem unnecessary to establish a free passage from the sinuses into the nose for drainage. The procedure had been by some considered an essential part of complete debridement in war injuries (STEWART and BOTTERELL, 1947).

Case 1.40. Depressed fracture of the frontal squama beneath a cut wound above the left eye, stitched up on admission. On the 3rd day, re-opening and debridement of a deep wound in left frontal lobe. Dural graft. Recovery.

A middle-aged Indian male was admitted with a superficially stitched-up cut wound above the left eye. There were no abnormal neurological signs. X-rays (Fig. 20) revealed a transverse fracture of the frontal squama crossing the midline just above the frontal sinus and running backwards into the temporal region.

A cluster of in-driven bones lay above and behind the frontal sinus which, as far as the radiological findings could be interpreted, was not involved.

Under local anaesthesia, the incision was re-opened and enlarged on the 3rd day after the injury. A fractured bone was exposed and it was found that the lower part of the frontal squama was somewhat loose. On nibbling away the bone edges along the fracture line a gap in the dura, size of a half-crown, was found, with bone fragments dislodged beneath the tabula interna as well as beneath the dura. Cerebrospinal fluid was leaking from the brain surface. There was a deep defect in the frontal lobe approximate size of a pigeon's egg, filled with debris, clotted blood, pulped brain and a number of small bone spicules. On cleansing the brain wound with

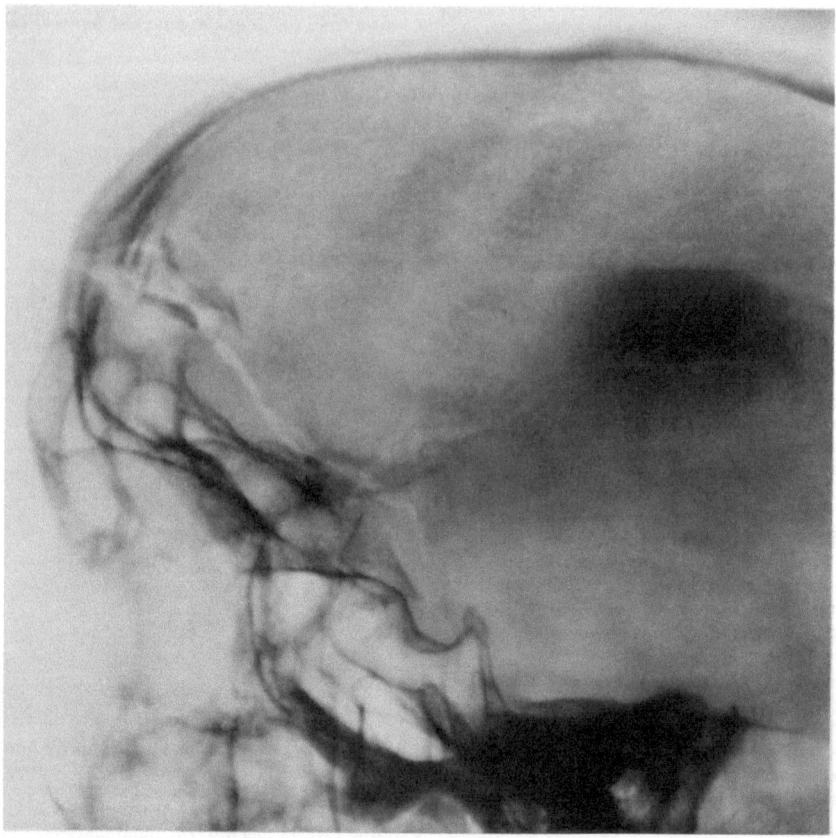

Fig. 20. X-ray of skull in a patient admitted with an open wound above the left eye which had been superficially stitched in the casualty service. Radiograph shows transverse fracture through frontal squama with in-driven bone chips. Although, on the films, the frontal sinus was not involved on exposure it was found full of blood clots. The sinus was exenterated including its mucosal lining. Primary closure after debridement of deep wound in left frontal lobe, and dural repair (Case 1.40)

the sucker, the falx and the superior sagittal sinus came into view in turn. In order to gain access to the base, the posterior wall of the frontal sinus was removed in toto; with this, it was found that the sinus was full of blood clots which were removed. The mucosa was rongeured away. There was no fracture in the floor of the anterior fossa. Haemostasis on the brain was completed with cautery, and a solution containing 20,000 units of penicillin was instilled into the brain wound. The dural tear was closed tightly with a pedicled graft from the epicranium and the dura hinged up to the periosteum. Sulphonamide powder was sprinkled onto the dura and the wound closed without drain in 2 layers. Quick and full recovery occurred and the wound healed primarily. The patient was discharged with a perfect scar overlying a slightly pulsating defect in the vault.

Comment. In this case, primary closure of a small scalp laceration above the left eye was carried out on admission before X-rays were taken which later showed a depressed fracture in close vicinity to the frontal sinus. Obviously, a careful exposure and inspection of the original wound would have disclosed the serious damage done to the dura mater as well as the brain. This failure of the first surgical attempt entailed re-opening of the wound on the 3rd day and final debridement of the deep structures with repair of the torn dura mater. This was followed by quick recovery.

Although, on the X-ray films, the frontal sinus itself was not involved in the fracture it turned out, on exposure, when its posterior wall was removed that the sinus was full of blood clots. Its complete exenteration was deemed necessary to eliminate any nidus of potential infection in so close a vicininy to a dural defect and a deep wound in the frontal lobe of the brain.

b) Standard incision (Osteoplastic flap)

It has been suggested as a routine procedure by ADSON (1941), R. C. SCHNEIDER and others to turn down a bilateral frontal flap and to ligate the sagittal sinus. We have not found this necessary in the majority of our cases since experience has shown that from a unilateral flap concealed within the hairline one gains satisfactory access to the cribriform plate and both orbital roofs. The tap of an aerocele or a dilated ventricle provides additional space and the brain collapsing like a deflated balloon in these cases allows viewing of the anterior fossa as far back as the sphenoidal ridge. This unilateral approach is similar to DANDY's standard incision for the exposure of the optic chiasm and the pituitary region (Fig. 21). In the following case a bilateral Souttard flap as suggested by SACHS (1925)[1] and TÖNNIS (1938, 1939) has been carried out and the superior sagittal sinus ligated to repair a bilateral frontal encephalocele.

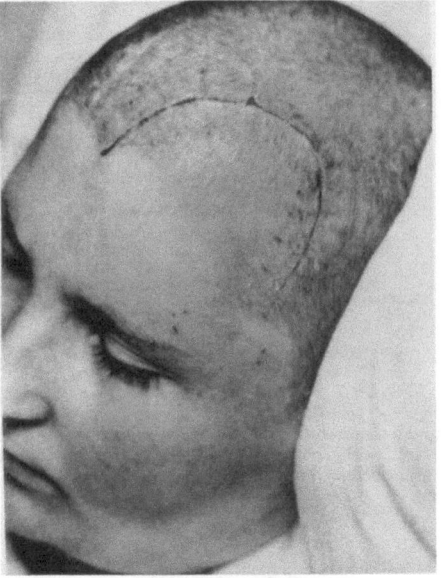

Fig. 21. To illustrate the standard incision for osteoplastic approach to the pituitary, optic chiasm, and cribriform plate, as developed by DANDY, OLIVECRONA and TÖNNIS. Appearance of scar on the 7th day after craniotomy. In most cases of fronto-basal injury requiring dural repair this unilateral flap is sufficient and gives access to the anterior fossa on both sides of the crista galli. Note marking out of the midline and small scar over the anterior horn on the opposite side for ventricular tap (if needed)

Case 1.15. African male of 14 with a tumour at the root of his nose thought to be a lipoma. Surgical attempt to remove it led to cerebrospinal fluid leakage. Bifrontal flap and removal of bilateral frontal encephalo-meningocele. Recovery.

On December 4th, 1987, an African boy, aged 14, was admitted on whom, in a district hospital, an operation had been performed in an attempt to remove what was thought to be a lipoma between his eyes. Soon it was incised, cerebrospinal fluid leakage occurred, surgery was abandoned, and the patient sent to the King Edward VIII Hospital in Durban. From the letter of the referring surgeon it was not clear whether a lipoma actually had been removed; at any rate, a pedunculated meningocele containing clear fluid was identified and found to extend through a defect in the region of the frontal sinus into the anterior cranial chamber. After this operation, off and on watery fluid escaped through the skin incision; however, no signs of actual meningitis developed. It was interesting to note that there was no mass protruding into the nasal meatus or nasopharynx, and, as far as could be ascertained, sensation of smell was present. The left eye showed a very slight protrusion and outward squint suggesting a bone defect in the roof of the left orbit. X-rays lent further support to this view. Otherwise, there were no neurological deviations and no other signs of dysraphism.

A bifrontal Souttard flap was raised and the sagittal sinus doubly ligated and cut between dural incisions. After reflecting the dura mater a pair of tongue-like extensions of either frontal pole came into sight stretching forward and downward, and occupying, on either side of the crista galli, a funnel-shaped defect in the anterior cranial fossa; it looked exactly like a bilateral cerebellar pressure cone. A fine picture of such frontal encephalocele, confined to the left side, is to be found on p. 56 of INGRAHAM and MATSON's *Neurosurgery of Infancy and Childhood* (1954). Fig. 22 illustrates the operative procedure in our case. As suggested by the X-rays the

---

[1] SACHS, E.: A method for exposing the anterior portion of the frontal lobes of the brain. Ann. Surg. **81**, 1053 (1925).

bone defect involving the medial parts of either orbital roof was much bigger on the left[1]. It was no easy task to disengage the herniated brain from its narrow meningocele sac. But we succeeded eventually in doing so without provoking a major bleeding. The two appendages of the frontal poles were then removed piece-meal and the defect in the anterior fossa packed with cancellous bone, that in the dura repaired with a free graft from the thigh fascia. Fig. 23 shows the boy at the time of discharge from the hospital.

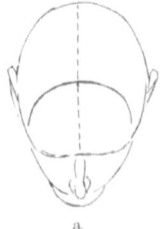

Fig. 22a—c. Featuring stages in operative repair of bilateral anterior encephalo-meningocele.

a bifrontal incision and right osteoplastic flap crossing the midline

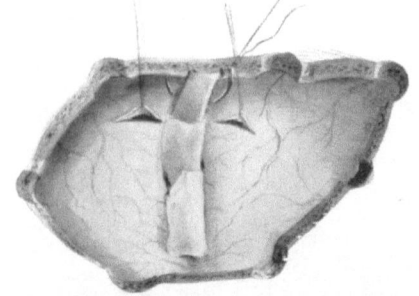

b dural incisions on either side of the sagittal sinus which is covered with cotton wool pledgets for haemostasis, and subsequently was ligated and severed

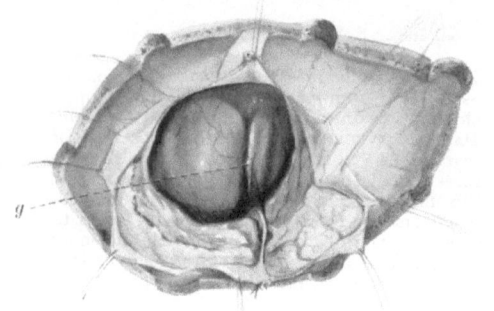

c the herniated brain has been removed on either side of the crista galli (g), the inside of the meningocele sac is exposed; it was much bigger on the left side than on the right in this case (Case 1.15)

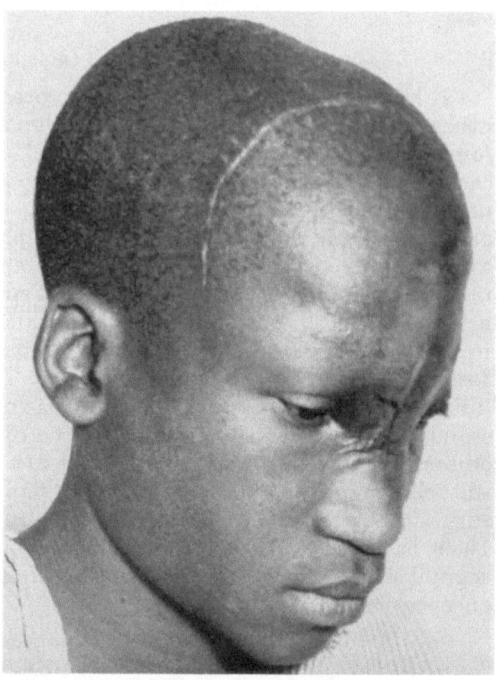

Fig. 23. Illustrating right half of operative scar in a case of bilateral anterior encephalomeningocele repaired by the intracranial approach as inaugurated by TÖNNIS (1939) in meningioma of the olfactory groove. Note stellate scar at root of nose indicating previous surgical attempt to remove a lipoma there; this had resulted in cerebro-spinal fluid leak (Case 1.15)

c) Dural repair

Search for the defect or defects in the dura will generally begin by the extradural approach on either side of the midline exposing the posterior wall of the frontal sinus, the cribriform plate and the orbital roofs; attempts to expose the sphenoidal sinus are difficult and usually unsuccessful. Multiple small tears in the dura are often found related to minute splinters of bone flung off the brittle posterior wall of the frontal sinus, the cribriform plate or even the crista galli. If too big to be stitched up by interrupted stitches the gaps in the dura have to be "patched up" by means of a free graft either from the

---

[1] DANDY, in his paper on carotid-cavernous aneurysms (1937), presents a drawing of congenital absence of the roof of the left orbit associated with absence of the cavernous sinus and the internal carotid artery on the same side. In his case details of which are not given by the author, the bone defect involved the minor sphenoidal wing and the adjacent portion of the left orbital roof. Absence of the ala minor on the left was suggested by the X-rays in our case.

fascia lata or — more conveniently — from the temporalis fascia or the pericranium; in the latter case a hinged flap is preferable. Large dural tears extending far back on the base of the skull often cannot be exposed and repaired in this way; it is then better to tuck in a fascial graft of adequate size between the dura and the floor of the anterior fossa, as exemplified by case 1.13 (p. 39), and to determine, by intradural inspection, whether the dural repair is watertight. This is facilitated by jugular compression after the dural closure has been completed.

In cases of extensive fissuring or defects in the orbital roof, orbital fat pushes into the cranial fossa and consequently has been used successfully to close a nearby dural defect as suggested by TÖNNIS, KRÜGER, SMALL and TURNER and others.

For dural defects near the midline KUHLENDAHL (1959) has advanced a "revolving" flap stripped off the dura covering the orbital roof similar to that the author (IRSIGLER, 1943) has used in cases of glioma of the optic nerve in order to replace the removed roof of the optic canal and to establish a protective barrier between the orbit and the basal cisterns. Also grafts from the falx cerebri, free and pedicled, have been suggested (GURD-JIAN and WEBSTER, 1944).

Not infrequently, and more so in cases of delayed surgical attack, herniated brain tissue will be found penetrating through a dural gap and plugging it entrapped, as it were, within a fracture or fissure in the base of the skull (case 1.8, p. 49). Adequate exposure of the dura over the convexity and along the floor of the anterior fossa implies removal of all completely loose bone. It is well.advised to nibble away the posterior wall of the frontal sinus whenever there is any doubt as to its being involved in order to inspect its interior. Most authors advise and, in fact, regard it essential to perform a complete ex-enteration, by way of suction or curettage, of the mucosal lining of the exposed sinuses so as to eradicate any source of potential infection which might endanger the dural repair and complicate the postoperative course. In cases where the mucosa of the frontal sinus was found intact and not bulging the author has left it untouched on several occasions without, as yet, any untoward sequelae. It would appear, then, to seal off the opening by a hinged graft from the nearby pericranium or temporalis fascia.

In the presence of comminuted fracture of the ethmoid plate as shown by X-rays or found on exposure it is essential to enlarge the debridement at this site to such extent as to establish a free draining passage into the upper nasal meatus as advocated by TÖNNIS (1941), KRÜGER (1942), STEWART and BOTTERELL, and others. Insertion of rubber drains issued through the nostrils was recommended by some authors at the beginning of the last war but later abandoned. With all the resources of present-day chemotherapy, local and systemic, this appears unnecessary, and may even be harmful.

For the same reason, the question of extradural, i.e. sub-aponeurotic drainage nowadays plays but a minor rôle; it is essential, however, to close the wound carefully without tension and, in case of necessity, by plastic flaps, using fine silk sutures for the pericranium and the skin.

7. Late manifestations

In what follows five common scquelae to fronto-basal injury will be described briefly and commented on to conclude each case history.
  a) Late frontal abscess.
  b) Recurrent cerebrospinal fistula.
  c) Frontal lobe atrophy.
  d) Late subdural aerocele in frontal region.
  e) Late frontogenous intracerebral aerocele.

a) Late frontal abscess

Case 1.4. Compound fronto-basal injury. Open wound above eye brows stitched up in the casualty service. Pneumococcal meningitis within 48 hours. Delayed radical debridement and wound closure. Healing by primary intention. Returned to work. — Death from left frontal abscess 21 months later.

The man whose face is shown in Fig. 24 was admitted to a general surgical ward with an open wound on his forehead, and a comminuted fracture involving both the frontal and the ethmoid sinuses. The casualty officer stitched up the wound superficially. Despite penicillin and sulphonamides, signs of meningitis became manifest clinically within the following 2 days; pneumococci were cultured from the lumbar fluid. There was no rhinorrhoea. The patient was now taken without further delay to the theatre and the fronto-basal area exposed by a cross-bow incision through both eye brows. The frontal sinus was shattered and full of blood clots and debris. There was a stellate fracture of its posterior wall which was removed, together with lose fragments from the ethmoid bone one of which had pierced through the dura resulting in a minute tear. This was closed

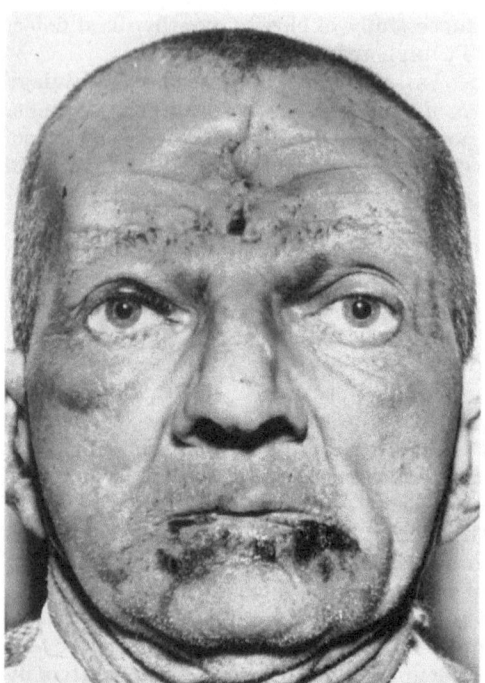

with a stitch and sealed off with gelatine foam. Then the wound was cleansed thoroughly and sulphonamide powder sprinkled into the pockets. Two soft rubber drains were issued on either side and the wound carefully closed up in layers. Speedy recovery without neurological deficit ensued. The wound healed practically per primary intention as shown in Fig. 24.

The man resumed his work as a gardener. Later on it was reported that troublesome personality changes had developed, obviously due to frontal lobe damage. One year and nine months later he was re-admitted to another ward but I was given the opportunity of seeing him again. He was lethargic and disorientated, and had a right hemiparesis and expressive aphasia. The surgical scar over his glabella was perfect and somewhat drawn in. There was no dural leak. It was obvious that a late frontal abscess had developed on the left side. At this stage a lumbar air encephalogram was attempted and resulted in deepening coma with unequivocal signs of tentorial coning. Unfortunately, operation was postponed and the patient died 5 days after admission. Autopsy revealed an old trephine opening in the frontal bone, and a brain abscess in the left frontal lobe. No meningitis was present.

Fig. 24. To illustrate cross bow (or "butterfly") incision after delayed surgical repair of a fronto-basal comminuted fracture. Note herpes labialis which had developed during attack of pneumococcal meningitis two days following injury; meningitis subsided after radical debridement and wound closure. The figure shows the patient at the time of his discharge from hospital. He died 21 months later from a late frontal lobe abscess without meningitis (Case 1.4)

Comment. Two points of importance are clearly demonstrated by this case. Firstly: a patient with local injury to his forehead involving the paranasal sinuses may develop an early meningeal infection even in the absence of a manifest dural leak, and despite chemotherapeutic "cover". This is evidenced still more conclusively in another patient in this series (case 1.26, p. 31). Superficial attention to a scalp laceration in the fronto-orbital region without wound cleansing and inspection of dura is ill-advised and creates a false confidence.

Secondly: once a patient has had an attack of meningitis, mild though it may be due to modern bacteriostatic and bactericidal agents, the clinician should be constantly and for a long time on the look-out for a late frontal abscess to be attacked without time-consuming and unnecessary diagnostic preliminaries. Behavioural deviations may be a significant clinical precursor and bridge over, as it were, the time gap between injury and the first symptoms indicative of intracranial infection. It is also noteworthy that a late frontal abscess, as in the above case, may present under a fulminating clinical picture characterized by fullblown signs of pressure cone.

Another remark seems called for here. In the presence of bouts of intracranial infection of seemingly obscure origin puzzling the diagnostic acumen of every surgeon, one should be aware of a neglected or long-forgotten injury to the paranasal sinuses; the situation here is somewhat similar to that in recurrent meningitic episodes due to a concealed pilonidal sinus.

b) Recurrent cerebrospinal fistula

Case 1.10. Recurrent rhinorrhoea on right side after dural repair with fascia. Advanced and progressive mental alteration. Tympanicity on percussion of right frontal region. Multi-loculated intracranial air cysts and spontaneous air encephalogram. Re-operation failed again.

This man, aged 42, had his post-traumatic, right-sided, rhinorrhoea which was associated with a frontal aerocele on the same side, repaired by means of a graft from the fascia lata. Four weeks later the cerebrospinal fistula recurred after an attack of headache, vomiting, and pyrexia. Neurologically, there was advanced mental dullness with double incontinence, anosmia on the right side with diminished smell sensation on the left, slight upper motor neuron facial weakness and increased tendon reflexes on the left. The optic discs were normal. On percussion of the right frontal area a conspicuous tympanicity was present. Plain X-rays of the skull revealed a pear-shaped aerocele occupying the right frontal lobe and communicating with the ventricular system. The anterior horns were both grossly dilated; in addition, a bilateral collection of air was present in the temporal fossae, probably within the subdural space. It was obvious, in comparing these pictures with those made previously, that the ventricular dilatation had increased considerably since.

A second attempt at dural repair was decided upon, five months after the first craniotomy. A right frontal osteoplastic flap was turned down again (Dr. G. WEBER) and the dura found firmly adherent to the brain over the convexity as well as at the base. Tap of the right ventricle yielded air at first, then clear fluid. The extradural approach along the orbital roof was now easy and led to exposure of defects both in the posterior wall of the right frontal sinus and in the cribriform plate; in the latter rather loose bony fragments surrounded the defect. The hole into the frontal sinus was much smaller. There was also a defect in the right orbital roof. Since all three bony openings were covered completely by intact dura mater, the impression was that leakage was not through one of the openings on the right. The floor of the anterior fossa to the left of the crista galli was visualised, too; no bone injury was found there. To be on the safe side, the three openings mentioned above were plugged with fascia lata and gelatine foam. The collapsed ventricles were then re-filled with 50 ml. of saline solution to which 20,000 units of penicillin had been added. The dura was closed tightly and hinged to the pericranium. The wound was closed in two layers. It healed per primary union. Plain X-rays taken on the 7th day following operation, disclosed a big aerocele over the frontal lobe on either side, the one on the right obviously being multilocular; in addition to this, the whole ventricular system including the 3rd and 4th ventricles, was outlined with air. Both frontal horns were distorted by the intra-cerebral aeroceles. From the 10th day onwards ample blood-stained discharge occurred from the right nostril in the patient when sitting upright. Aspiration through one of the trephine openings yielded air only. Within 45 seconds after instillation of 2,5 ml. of indigo carmine the dye appeared from the right nostril. On rhinoscopy the blue path of leakage could be traced upwards into the region of the cribriform plate. On discharge from the clinic, the patient's mental and neurological set-up was virtually the same as before the operation.

Comment. In view of the operative findings a leakage through the sphenoid sinus was considered a possibility. However, in retrospect and also on the ground of the postoperative rhinoscopic appearance it would seem more likely that the double recurrence of the cerebrospinal fistula occurred through the defect in the right cribriform plate which, on exposure, had revealed a comminuted fracture. Possibly, the lesson to be learned from this experience is that, in the presence of a shattered ethmoid bone radical removal of all loose bone fragments including the cribriform plate should be carried out as a routine procedure prior to dural repair at this site.

It may be debatable whether, with regard to the progressive mental deterioration reducing the patient to hardly more than a vegetative state further surgical attempts are justifiable.

c) Atrophy of frontal lobes

Case 1.9. Meningo-cerebral scarring and atrophy of right frontal lobe with old haemorrhagic cavities associated with indriven bone chips and intracerebral aerocele in chronic cerebrospinal fistula via the right frontal sinus. Successful repair.

Only the pertinent data will be given. This man, 34 of age, presented with a right-sided rhinorrhoea. He was admitted for operation to the Neurosurgical Clinic in Zürich. On elevating a right frontal osteoplastic flap (Prof. H. KRAYENBÜHL) a depressed fracture of the frontal bone was exposed. The dura mater was slack. The brain convolutions were flattened. Marked respiratory movements of the brain were noticed conveying the impression of a blow-pipe in action and indicating a large intracerebral air cyst. As the dura was adherent to the brain surface an extra-dural approach was decided upon. On stripping the dura from the floor of the anterior fossa a stellate fracture of the right orbital roof came into sight. The dura was trapped between the fragments. In the middle of a large meningo-encephalitic scar, adherent to the posterior wall of the frontal sinus, a hole, size of a pea, in the latter was exposed and plugged with wax and gelatine foam. A corresponding defect in the dura was closed with a free graft from the thigh fascia. After incision of the dura an extensive area of infarction on the base of the right frontal lobe came into view; the devitalized brain substance was of a peculiar yellowish tinge and contained numerous small haemorrhagic cysts and, in addition, an in-driven bone splinter lodging near the falx cerebri; evidently, this piece of bone came from the posterior wall of the frontal sinus. On dissecting the fragment from the surrounding tissue a smooth-walled intracerebral air cyst was opened. The subdural space now was re-filled with saline solution; no fluid escaped from the nose. This was taken as indicating a water-tight dural repair. 15,000 units of penicillin were instilled subdurally and the dura was hinged up to the pericranium. The flap was re-sutured in layers.

The patient was discharged without signs of recurrence and reported full working capacity as a farmer seven months later.

Comment. Such procedure as carried out in the above case may be time-consuming but as the result has shown, may be gratifying even in the presence of frontal lobe damage. One would expect, and it had been confirmed in war injuries that bone fragments dislodged intradurally are likely to be associated with corresponding atrophic and cystic degeneration of the brain substance, especially the orbital and medial surfaces of the frontal lobes.

The combined extradural and intradural approach appears to be the procedure of choice in similar cases complicated by extensive meningo-cerebral scarring.

d) Late subdural aerocele in frontal region

Case 1.38. Localized atrophy of the left frontal lobe associated with a subdural aerole which developed-following lumbar air encephalograpy eleven months after blunt injury to the fronto-orbital region which had resulted in surgical emphysema around the left eye.

On admission, this 31-year-old man gave the history of a dizzy spell followed, the same night, by intense occipital headache. It was learned that some eleven months previously, he had suffered a knock against his forehead which had resulted in a surgical emphysema of the upper lid of his left eye. Air was aspirated whereupon the eye lid went down "like a pricked balloon". Since no discharge from his nose was noted nor were there any complaints on the part of the patient no X-rays were taken at the time.

On admission now, eleven months after that incident, examination revealed normal fundi and, except for a suggestion of weakness of his right arm, no neurological deviations. A left carotid angiogram disclosed a considerable spill of the dye across the midline and into the right sylvian group; on the a-p. view, there was no shift but some local distortion of both anterior cerebral arteries. The venous phase demonstrated one of the ascending veins in a peculiar way straightened out. The over-all impression was that of some local pathology in the left frontal region. Subsequently, air was instilled by the lumbar route. The fluid was clear and under normal pressure. The films showed no definite shift across the midline; however, in none of the views taken, the left anterior horn was clearly visualised. Following these diagnostic procedures which were carried out under general anaesthesia the patient failed to come around swiftly and the following night became restless and delirious; he climbed out of his bed, soiled his night dress and was found lying on the floor. A right-sided hemiplegia was now apparent. He remained in a state of clouded consciousness with obvious difficulty in speaking and understanding what he was told. There were no signs of raised intracranial pressure, and the pupils were equal and with brisk reaction to light. The blood pressure was slightly elevated all the time. By the next morning, the power on his right side had recovered slightly but the patient remained drowsy and aphasic; he took his feeds well. It was felt that this might be either a carotid thrombosis or a deep-seated left frontal mass. The same day the patient developed a series of epileptic convulsions merging into status epilepticus which was cut short by intravenous barbiturate. A left temporo-frontal flap was now turned down under general anaesthesia. Cutting the bone with the GIGLI saw made a striking "hollow" sound. The dura was slack, even wrinkled. Underneath it there was a shifting fluid level visible and palpable; this air bag, size of a peach approximately, occupied the anterior and lateral parts of the frontal cortex. On incising the dura cerebrospinal fluid escaped freely from the subdural aerocele. The presenting frontal lobe revealed a normal convolutional pattern; an ascending cortical vein came into view, its stretched course and dichotomy corresponding exactly to the phlebogram as reported above. A fair amount of cerebrospinal fluid escaped also from the subarachnoid pathways over the convexity so that the mesial aspect of the left hemisphere could easily be brought into sight by retracting the frontal lobe. On gentle palpation of the cortex surrounding the vein just mentioned an impression of abnormal softness was gained; needling met with no pathological resistance. A cortical incision was carried down through this area revealing a diffuse rubber-like gliosis of the brain. A number of small pieces of tissue were excised for biopsy; neither a tumour nor a cyst was encountered. The resulting "crater" in the brain was lined with oxycel for haemostasis. The wound was closed in the usual layers. Recovery was quick and complete. The patient was discharged without neurological deficit. Histology of the excised tissue showed gliosis with local increase in microglia and small fresh haemorrhages due to the operation. No signs of a neoplasm were found.

Comment. If our interpretation of the sequence of events in this case was right it must be assumed that a blunt injury to the fronto-orbital region such as to produce a surgical emphysema may also be severe enough so as to result in a localized brain atrophy in the adjacent frontal lobe. We do not know, of course, whether, following the injury, an intracranial aerocele was present in the left anterior fossa wihthout making symptoms; if so, it could have been a contributing factor to the atrophic changes in the underlying frontal lobe.

Since a subdural collection of air was not shown on the encephalogram nor found on exposure it follows that this was a condition of quite recent origin related to the air insufflation forming what could be called a factitious aerocele. Perhaps, a predisposing factor to its development and rapid expansion was the atrophic shrinkage of the brain tissue beneath as indicated by the dilated subarachnoid pathways.

It is noteworthy that the air cyst grew so rapidly to a space-occupying mass as to make, within a few hours, severe neurological symptoms related to the pre-rolandic and BROCA's convolutions — a feature, to be sure, which is well-known from intracerebral aeroceles arising by a sudden rise in pressure such as induced by coughing and sneezing. Craniotomy, in our case, resulted in evacuation of the intracranial air followed by fast and complete recovery of the patient. A vascular lesion of recent origin as well as a late frontal abscess had to be considered in differential diagnosis; both were ruled out by the appearance to the naked eye and microscopy.

e) Late frontogenous intracerebral aerocele

Case 1.8. Left frontal craniotomy in a man of 23 with an intracerebral aerocele due to fronto-basal injury 9 weeks previously. Fissuring of the lamina cribriformis. Traumatic brain hernia. Intradural approach and grafting. Recovery.

This man fell from a bicycle and remained unconscious for two hours. A laceration above the left eye brow was stitched up in a nearby hospital and the patient sent home. On the 2nd day after the accident a watery

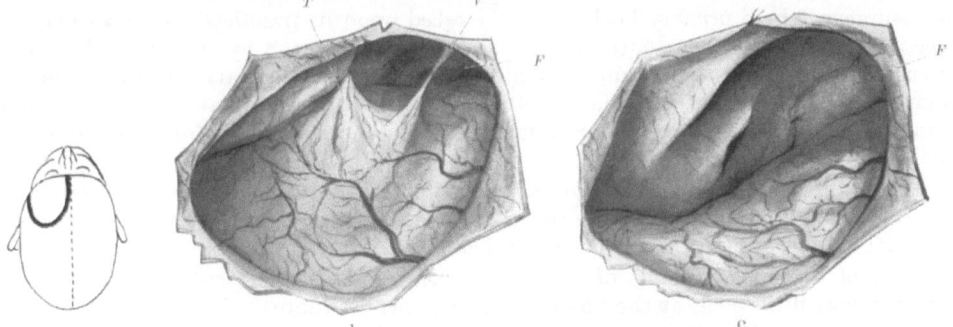

Fig. 25a—c. Featuring stages in operative approach to intracerebral aerocele following fracture of the cribriform plate on the left side (Case 1.8).   a Incision of scalp.   b The aerocele has been emptied by tap, and collapsed. A thin layer of cerebral cortex is anchored to the falx cerebri (F) by a bridging vein (V) and by being trapped (T) between fragments of the ethmoid bone.   c Left frontal lobe retracted to show more clearly the fractured ethmoid and exposed part of the falx.
(Drawing by Mr. H. P. WEBER, Neurosurgical University Clinic in Zürich)

discharge from the left nostril was noted but subsided within the ensuing few days. Five weeks later, a neurologist saw the man and noticed a peculiar splashing noise on shaking the patient's head. X-rays revealed a fracture line traversing the left frontal squama and an intracranial aerocele, size and shape of a hen's egg, occupying the left frontal area. The patient complained of anosmia on the left and progressing failure of vision in the left eye; there was a primary atrophy of the left optic disc.

Under local anaesthesia a left frontal osteoplastic flap was turned down from the standard incision behind the air line (Fig. 25). There was a fracture on the inner table of the bone flap. The dura mater was rather tense; it was hinged up to the pericranium and "nicked". A brain cannula was then inserted and hit a subcortical cavity from which 1 fl. oz. (about 30 ccm.) of clear yellow fluid were aspirated. The dura now slackened down, and was incised and reflected. The brain had collapsed, too, but was hinged, as it were, to the sagittal sinus by several cortical veins bridging the subdural space. They were carefully spared. On lifting up the frontal pole patchy adhesions were found between the brain surface and the dura on the base. They were severed. The pia-arachnoid there had a yellowish tinge. The posterior wall of the frontal sinus was intact. There was a fracture in the cribriform plate next to the crista galli and brain was herniating through the dura being intrapped between the bone fragments. Apparently it was at this site that the dural leak into the nose had taken place after the injury. A circumscribed contused area was exposed over the base of the brain involving the whole of the left olfactory region. The left optic nerve and sylvian group were found intact (obviously, the left optic nerve had been damaged within the optic canal). The structures on the right side were normal. The patient now was asked to strain by forcible expiration; no air or fluid leak occurred nor did the collapsed brain expand upon this manoeuvre. A doubled-up graft from the thigh fascia was taken and spread out so as to cover the whole of the left anterior fossa; it was then sutured to the inner surface of the dura and to the falx cerebri with interrupted silk. Haemostasis and water-tight closure of the dura followed. The wound was closed in the usual way. The patient stood the operation which had lasted $2^{1}/_{2}$ hours very well and recovered quickly; unfortunately, no details of the patient's convalescence are available.

The local anaesthesia had been satisfactory throughout thus confirming our previous impressions in war injuries to the effect that patients with fronto-basal injuries requiring a delicate and often time-consuming surgical intervention, tolerate local anaesthesia much better than general anaesthesia (vide p. 51). During debridement of the ethmoid region and twisting out the mucosal lining of the sinuses a small amount of evipan or pentothal may be needed to supplement the local anaesthetic.

8. War injuries

Here, as in accident wounds, the outstanding problem is prevention of intracranial spread of infection; in fact, the advances in management of war injuries since 1914 can best be gauged by the drop in incidence of severe intracranial infections: whereas in CUSHING's series of 1918, there were 31% of fulminating and fatal intracranial infections the percentage during the last war fell to 15% (CAIRNS, 1947) and even less[1]. Owing to the adopted principles of early and complete debridement, primary closure of dura and scalp, and chemotherapy, healing per primary union of war injuries to the skull was achieved in 75 to 85% of cases on either side of the World War II frontiers (GULEKE, 1940[2]; SMALL and TURNER, 1947). This approximates well to accident wounds in civilian neurosurgery where primary healing can be relied upon in practically all cases even irrespective of time of surgical intervention as it is demonstrated by the groups III and IV discussed above. It is important to realize, however, that primary healing of the scalp wound does not rule out early meningitis from treated and untreated wounds becoming manifest clinically as early as 48 hours following injury to the fronto-basal area, in civilian and war injuries alike.

It is in the very nature of high velocity missile wounds involving the paranasal cavities that makes them considerably more susceptible to contamination quickly followed by bacterial invasion and intracranial extension of infection.

First of all, most wounds of this type open up a straightforward avenue into the cerebrospinal fluid pools at the base of the brain; consequently, a direct infection of the leptomeninges is the rule even in cases where a basal meningitis develops only after some delay due to the dural tear being plugged temporarily by swelling or devitalized brain tissue (CAIRNS, 1947). This mode of meningial infection is essentially different from that following wounds on the convexity where, owing to early occlusion of subdural and subarachnoid pathways (ATKINSON, SPATZ) around the entrance into the brain, the infection reaches the meninges commonly by spreading along the track within the brain tissue (CAIRNS, 1937) eventually to reach the ventricles, and resulting in an "indirect" type of meningitis.

Furthermore, the opening-up of the paranasal sinuses including the orbital roof extension of the frontal sinus in unsuspected fissuring of this lamellar part of the floor of the anterior fossa (SPATZ, JOHNSON and DUTT, KLAUE) is likely to provide an additional nidus of infection, be it pre-existent or due to bacterial invasion from outside or to upper respiratory embarrassement. Dormant infection of the accessory air cavities not dealt with adequately during the first surgical attempt, has been found to account for the majority of intracranial infective complications, such as extradural abscesses, subdural empyemas between the hemispheres and at the base of the brain, as well as cerebral abscesses opposite to a strictly unilateral path of the missile; the same possibly applies to thrombosis and thrombophlebitis of the superior sagittal sinus. Some of these features will be exemplified later by case histories (case 1.3 and 1.7).

---

[1] During the Korean campaign MEIROWSKY and HARSH reported less than 1% meningo-cerebral infections in penetrating head wounds (1959).
[2] Dtsch. Mil.arzt **5**, 93 (1940).

Early obstruction of the air passages is facilitated by complicated wounds involving the mouth, jaws, pharynx and larynx not uncommon in through-and-through missile wounds of the face and neck.

Indriven and often far-dislodged bony fragments and foreigns bodies encountered in high velocity missile wounds indicate the more extensive damage to the dura mater and the brain with consequent accumulation of pulped, non-viable brain tissue, bacterial pabulum and purulent collections in the missile tracks often difficult to trace, especially in ricochet wounds.

Finally, hypothalamic involvement inherent in all kinds of injury to the base of the skull, is obviously per se responsible for the prognosis in some cases. Damage to the brain stem is indicated by clinical signs of brain swelling (JOHNSON and DUTT) such as early and persistent or progressive lowering of the conscious level with suppression of the cough and pharyngeal reflexes followed by obstructed air passages which inter alia makes the diagnosis of a concealed cerebrospinal fluid leak a difficult matter. Circulatory and postural hypotension is a well-known feature of hypothalamic impairment be it traumatic or with tumours lodging at this site (TÖNNIS, 1950; CAUGHEY and GARROD, 1954).

The two case histories which conclude the present chapter, both from the early years of World War II and for this reason somewhat lacking in detail, will serve to illustrate, from a practical point of view, some of the points raised above.

Surgical management

a) Anaesthesia

Whenever possible local anaesthesia should be given preference and supplemented if necessary e.g. on debriding deep structures, by small amounts of a short-acting barbiturate.

b) Approach

No general agreement was reached during the last war, and probably no rigid rules can be laid down under the conditions prevailing during war, as to the best type of approach for surgical repair of fronto-basal injuries, whether by direct route i.e. enlarging the bone defect of the original wound, or by a formal osteoplastic flap "from above". The direct route at the site of entry combined with radical exenteration of the paranasal sinuses was generally given preference at the beginning of the last war, and it would appear that this is the most suitable procedure under the stress of the battlefield and in all cases where lacerations of the scalp are such as to require per se an immediate and more elaborate surgical intervention providing adequate access for inspection of the dura on either side of the midline. In most cases it was found necessary to enlarge the original wound by additional incisions along the eye brows or in the midline, or even to make a unilateral or bilateral hinged forehead flap. The more common types of incisions have been repeatedly described (IRSIGLER, 1960). Later in the war, with the dural repair becoming recognized more and more as of paramount importance, and with the facilities provided by air evacuation, the intradural approach by standard incisions and osteoplastic flap came into more general use especially among the British neurosurgeons (CAIRNS, 1947; CALVERT, 1947). It is the procedure of choice in all cases of delayed surgical intervention when the original wound is already healed up or has been closed successfully by early operation; it may then still be a problem of intricate plastic repair.

c) Management of the exposed sinuses

Whereas removal of completely loose or too heavily contaminated bone, especially the walls of the sinuses, is, to a certain degree, a matter of opinion, there is fairly general consensus as to the radical exenteration of the involved air cavities including clot and debris as well as the mucosa lining their inner surface (TÖNNIS, 1941; KRÜGER, 1943; SMALL and TURNER, 1947; STEWART and BOTTERELL, 1947). This principle of radical debridement should be adhered to irrespective of the immediate cosmetic result; sparing as much as possible of the super-ciliary arch of the frontal bone greatly facilitates later reconstruction. With regard to the ethmoid sinus and cribriform plate, thorough wound cleansing most often results in establishing a free passage into the upper nasal meatus which provides adequate drainage into the nose; the importance of the latter procedure is stressed even by those authors advising against stripping of the mucosa which may result, according to them, in unnecessary bleeding (JOHNSON and DUTT, 1947). Inadequate debridement at the site of the ethmoid may well imply recurrent dural leak as exemplified by the case 1.10 in the present series reported above (p. 47).

d) Cleansing of the missile track

Following a missile track in the brain and careful removal, mostly by gentle suction, of all devitalized or diffluent tissue, debris, foreigns bodies, and clot, is essential to eliminate any source of smouldering infection and to prevent early purulent retention and late abscess. This stage of the operation may well be a time-consuming procedure, especially in ricochet and through-and-through wounds. To perform this properly a narrow, malleable, and possibly lighted brain rectractor is most useful and, in fact, no less indispensable than an efficient suction apparatus.

e) Dural repair

Inspection and repair of the torn dura is considerably facilitated by any degree of intracranial hypotension; TÖNNIS (1941) has suggested pre-operative lumbar puncture to lower the pressure. Dural repair may be a difficult task during the acute stage after wounding complicated by oedema of the frontal lobes; it may even be technically impracticable to expose a large dural tear in its entire extent; a free fascial graft large enough to be doubled up at the sites not easily accessible, and tucked in loosely between the brain and the laid open sinuses, as well as use of mobilized orbital tissue as suggested by TÖNNIS, KRÜGER, SMALL and TURNER and many others, will provide the required protective barrier to minimize the risk of intradural spread of infection and of cerebrospinal fistula; an accident case of similar type has been described above (case 1.13, p. 39). Sealing off a communication to the sinus merely by wax or gelatine foam, or even with muscle, has proved inadequate. Intradural inspection will assist greatly in carrying out the dural repair with appropriate safety and should not be neglected whenever the dura mater has been incised. Finally, leakage through the sphenoid sinus not amenable to surgical repair, or through an unsuspected fissure in the petrous bone should be considered a remote possibility in rare instances.

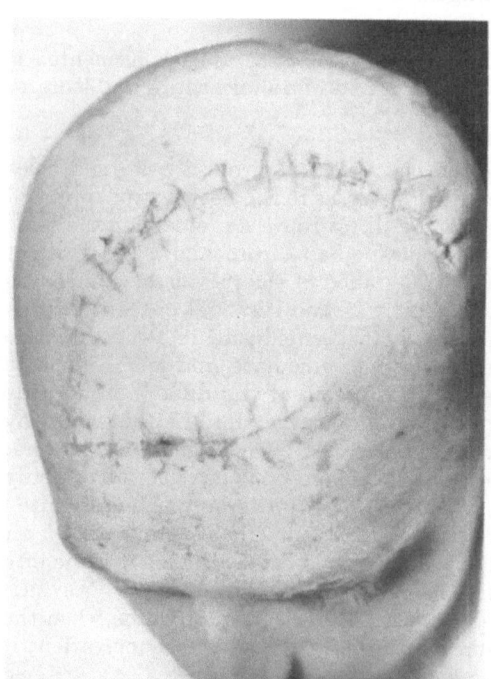

Fig. 26. To illustrate primary wound closure by means of a sliding flap in a patient with a penetrating bullet wound and loss of scalp on the forehead

f) Closure of scalp

If there is extensive tissue loss in the fronto-orbital area plastic manoeuvres become necessary in order to achieve primary closure in two layers and without undue tension to the stitches. Here, a truly gratifying field of plastic surgery was opened up during the last war. In general, tripod incisions of the scalp, as advocated originally by CUSHING are better replaced by sliding or rotating flaps of the S-type such as illustrated in Fig. 26. The advantages of primary and complete closure of the scalp wound were recognized early in the last war; it helps to keep the dural graft viable and tight, it prevents or at least minimizes secondary infection and brain herniation resulting in further destruction of brain tissue; finally, it facilitates greatly postoperative care saving much time and dressings.

g) Drainage

The insertion of small tubes or slivers of rubber beneath the skin flap for extradural drainage was thought essential, and probably rightly so, before the penicillin era; even nowadays, it is still recommended in the management of fronto-basal injuries (KUHLEN-DAHL, 1959). It is hardly doubtful that this sort of drainage if not done with due care may facilitate secondary infection and disruption of the dural barrier thus becoming "a source of danger rather than of safety" (JEFFERSON, 1947); however my own experiences have tought that soft rubber tubes of the Penrose type do no harm if issued through button holes or small counter incisions outside the main wound and if removed after 24 to 48 hours while the patient is still under systemic chemotherapy, provided the dural repair has been adequate, the haemostasis perfect, and the closure done in two layers with careful stitches to the epicranium.

Management in the forward area

To a certain degree this must remain controversial since no general rules can be laid down applicable to changing conditions of any future war (OGILVIE, 1944). However, it is generally agreed that the type of missile wounds under consideration should be attacked surgically — however trifling the approach may be — at such places in the forward area only where appropriate X-ray and operative facilities including a suction apparatus are available, and where the wounded can stay in safety until all signs of any type of shock have subsided. It should be stressed that primary closure of dura and scalp may require high technical skill and special equipment. During World War II, evacuation by air has increasingly made up for the time-lag in reception and opened up new horizons regarding early and final debridement by fully equipped neurosurgical teams, on both sides of the frontiers.

It should be pressed on any surgeon called upon to attend first to an open brain wound that on him and his actions to a very great extent depends what will eventually become of the wound and of the wounded (KENNETH EDEN, 1944); even the most modern chemotherapy cannot compensate for inadequate primary surgery. Going into some details the following points seem worth mentioning:

A preliminary lumbar puncture will facilitate the approach and viewing the operative field. The operative intervention, then, should be by the direct route as exemplified in the two case histories 1.4 and 1.13 (pp. 45 and 39 respectively) presented above, and should include: 1. Debridement of the wound, superficial and deep, of all layers in turn, according to accepted surgical principles; 2. Establishing the diagnosis of dural involvement; this is essential for the follow-up of the case; a short note to this effect, together with a sketch of neurological findings made on the case sheet accompanying the wounded has proved most useful in the British Army; it has been also practised, to my knowledge, in the German Luftwaffe. 3. Repair of the torn dura mater should be restricted to extradural manoeuvres using free or pedicled graft from fascia, orbital tissue, or pericranium. Meticulous haemostasis to prevent residual clots must always be attempted though a diathermy apparatus and silver clips will not always be available in the forward area. Gelatine film can safely be replaced by hammered muscle. 4. Closure of the scalp should be complete and final and without tension, in two layers, using plastic procedures and relaxation incisions freely; resulting raw surfaces may be packed loosely or if time allows covered with

THIERSCH grafts. It is debatable whether during the first week repeated lumbar taps should be done in order to lower tension on the stitches. TÖNNIS, with good reasons, has advised against this manoeuvre.

To summarize the negative points: In the forward area no operative intervention however trifling should be attempted without X-rays of the skull. No osteoplastic cranio-tomies should be performed. Intradural manoeuvres should be avoided or restricted to cleansing the subdural space, and to indispensable haemostasis. Primary cranioplasty is not recommended.

Case 1.3. Penetrating missile wound through left fronto-basal area. Incomplete debridement in advanced field unit followed by incarcerated cerebral fungus which persisted after second surgical intervention 20 days after wounding, and recurred despite repeated lumbar punctures. Re-exploration 9 days thereafter. Interhemi-spherical empyema evacuated and drained. On decapping the cerebral fungus an abscess in the left frontal lobe was found and drained. Death 6 weeks after wounding. Autopsy: Left frontal lobe abscess and purulent meningitis over convexity and on the base extending between the cerebral hemispheres.

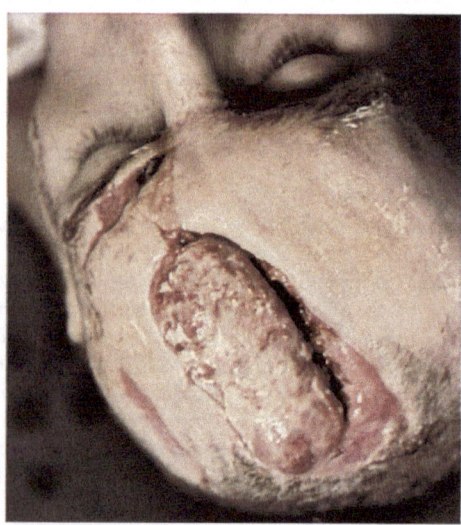 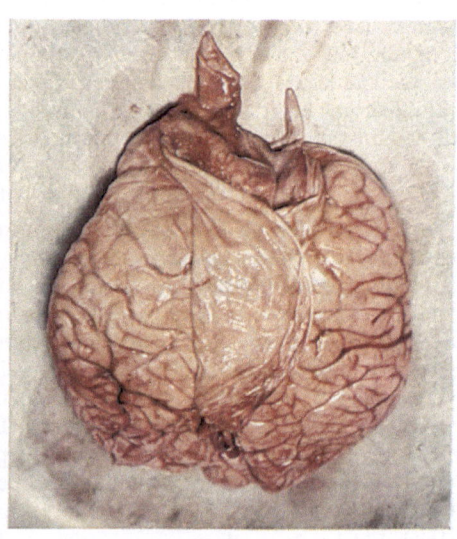

Fig. 27   Fig. 28

Fig. 27. Incarcerated encephalitic prolaps on the forehead following missile wound through left frontal sinus. Condition 20 days after injury. Two unsuccessful surgical attempts had been made. Underlying the fungating mass, there was an abscess in the left frontal lobe. Despite decapping of the fungation and drainage of the abscess, the patient died 6 weeks after wounding from purulent meningitis extending between the hemispheres (Case 1.3)

Fig. 28. Necropsy specimen of the patient shown in preceding figure, to illustrate walled-off abscess in left frontal lobe following penetrating missile wound through frontal sinus. The dura mater has been reflected to show purulent meningitis over left hemisphere (Case 1.3). (From the Institute of Pathology, Charité in Berlin)

This young soldier had sustained a small-missile wound penetrating through the left frontal sinus. He had received superficial attention in a forward echelon; no details of this surgical attempt were available. When admitted to the neurosurgical Clinic, nearly 3 weeks after wounding (Fig. 27), a big cerebral fungus had devel-oped occupying the mid-frontal region and showing signs of incarceration at its neck owing to a trephine opening which was too narrow to allow for adequate exposure and dural repair. Although the surface of the fungus was covered in part with granulations, there were no pulsations and a marked cyanosis. Lumbar taps failed to reduce the hernia in size. Furthermore, it was found on re-exploration that the anterior as well as the posterior walls of the frontal sinus were shattered and bone fragments had been left behind. What was left of the sinus cavity was now occupied by the cerebral herniation. A big plug of gauze had been put in alongside the sinus in a vain attempt to keep the wound open and to allow for drainage and closure per secundam. Instead, the cerebral fungus of unusual size shown in Fig. 27 had developed and, in its turn, aggravated the obstruction.

Secondary debridement with enlargment of the trephine opening, together with repeated lumbar punctures brought the herniation back almost to skin level. The lumbar fluid, at that time, was clear and colourless, with normal protein and cell count. However, the cerebral hernia recurred soon, even after ventricular tap, carried out over both posterior horns; it yielded but a few ml. of fluid, obviously too little to provide any relief of pressure. Attacks of meningitis made the patient increasingly drowsy and caused rise in temperature and profuse sweating. In his lucid intervals the patient showed pronounced mental derangement indicating serious frontal lobe damage. No rhinorrhoea was present, nor any cerebrospinal fluid leak from the wound.

On the 9th day after admission, a purulent collection was evacuated from the interhemispherical space and drained with a soft rubber drain. On decapping the fungus, a chronic, well-encapsulated abscess in the left frontal lobe was exposed and drained. Subsequently, although there was ample purulent discharge from the wound, drainage proved to be inadequate and pent-up pus had to be sucked off repeatedly from behind the prolaps and from the abscess cavity which, following a second decapping, was "opened up" and was found to be lined by a layer of fresh granulations.

Following an intervening erysipelas of the face with bullous eruptions the cerebral herniation occurred again and caused anew complete obstruction. A generous lumbar tap was now performed following which the prolapse receded beneath skin level, thus opening up the abscess cavity to form a deep crater with purulent retention within. The sudden relief of pressure was followed by progressive drowsiness, overbreathing and profuse sweating with rapid pulse and pyrexia. The patient succumbed the following night, nearly 6 weeks after wounding.

Necropsy revealed a well walled-off abscess cavity occupying the greater part of the left frontal lobe (Fig. 28) with widespread oedema of the left hemisphere and a purulent meningitis of comparatively recent origin and spreading over the convexity as well as the base of the brain; it extended also into the interhemispherical fissure, without, however, there causing a purulent retention of surgical proportions.

Comment. The ill effects of inadequate primary surgery are clearly demonstrated in the above case which, as every experienced neurosurgeon will agree, stands for many others seen in civilian and military service alike. Failure to obtain primary union and incomplete removal of indriven bone fragments, all too frequently spell the vicious circle of cerebral herniation, abscess, and meningitis (KENNETH EDEN, 1944). Surgical attempts at a later stage with established intra-dural infection are not infrequently unsuccessful because of the difficulty in drainage to be carried out in time and constantly secured. It is open to debate whether in our case radical excision of the encapsulated frontal abscess would have changed the course, in view of the early development of a large empyema between the two hemispheres. At any rate, decapping of a chronic cerebral hernia has been found ill-advised by others (SCHWARZ and ROULHAC, 1945). Repeated lumbar taps often fail to reduce the intracranial pressure persistently if not carried out judiciously; moreover, they even may spell the dangers of pressure fluctuations and bouts of meningitis which, in cases of fronto-basal injury and with the path of missile strictly, unilateral, may involve both hemispheres.

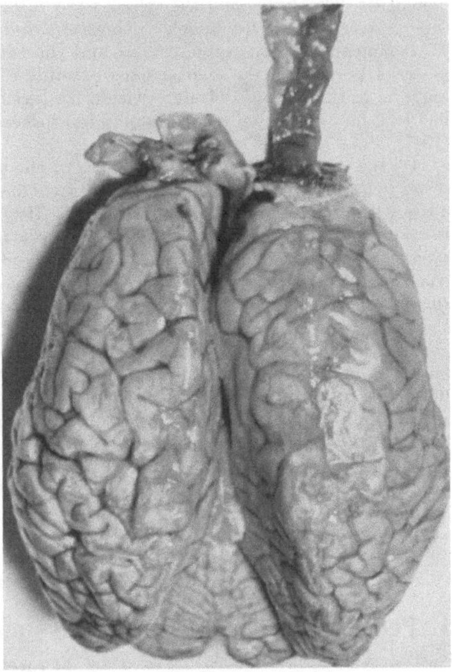

It is also significant that in the notes available from the above case there is no mentioning of sulphonamide

Fig. 29. Necropsy specimen from the Institute of Pathology (Professor R. RÖSSLE) of the Charité-Krankenhaus in Berlin. Purulent thrombophlebitis of the superior sagittal sinus extending into right lateral sinus and nearby cortical veins. Death occurred four weeks after missile wound through forehead followed by cerebral fungus. Note oedema of the right cerebral hemisphere indicating unsuspected abscess in the right rolandic region. An abscess in the right frontal lobe had been drained one week before death (Case 1.7)

drugs which possibly indicates that at that time (1941) they were used without much confidence in many cases.

Case 1.7. Small-missile wound through forehead followed by necrotising cerebral fungus. Drainage of early abscess in right frontal lobe 3 weeks after wounding. Staphylococcal meningitis. Left-sided hemiparesis progressing from face to leg. Lethargy. Death 4 weeks after wounding. Autopsy: Right frontal abscess. Purulent thrombophlebitis in posterior part of sagittal sinus extending into right lateral sinus and cortical veins. Cortical abscess in right rolandic region near the midline.

This 32-year-old soldier had sustained a small-missile wound in the middle of his forehead and was admitted 15 days after wounding with a pedicled cerebral fungus the superficial parts of which were necrotic. X-rays showed a cluster of indriven bone fragments. Re-exploration 3 weeks after wounding revealed a multilocular abscess cavity in the right frontal lobe containing thick pus. A soft rubber drain was inserted and the edges of the incision approached by scalp sutures. Two days later staphylococci were cultured from a clear and colourless lumbar fluid. The following day weakness of the left half of the face was noted. The scalp overlying the trephine opening was sunk. The hemiparesis progressed steadily to involve the left leg and arm but with the leg more affected. There was a fair amount of purulent discharge from the drain and again staphylococci were found in a smear and on culture from the drain. On removing the drain a narrow track could be seen leading into the abscess cavity whose bottom lay approximately 8 cm. from the surface. There was no cerebrospinal fluid leak. The man died 4 weeks after injury.

Necropsy was carried out by Professor R. Rössle. He found a big abscess in the right frontal lobe surrounded by an area of brain oedema, as indicated by flattened convolutions (Fig. 29). There was a middle-sized cortical abscess already shut off by dural adhesions in the right rolandic area near the midline. This abscess obviously was the result of retrograde cortical thrombophlebitis. Finally, there was a purulent thrombosis, not quite recent in origin and occupying the posterior third of the sagittal sinus; it extended into the right lateral and sigmoid sinuses both of which were obliterated. There was also a retrograde thrombophlebitis in some of the veins on the convexity draining into the thrombosed part of the sagittal sinus. The lateral sinus on the left was patent and so were the anterior $^2/_3$ of the superior longitudinal sinus. There were no signs of meningitis. The lungs and the spleen were normal. There was an incipient pachymeningitis haemorrhagica interna over the left frontal lobe with recent and somewhat older haemorrhages.

Comment. The interesting feature and the cause of death in this case was a septic thrombophlebitis of the posterior portion of the sagittal sinus extending into and obstructing the right lateral sinus. There were no sequelae to this thrombophlebitis within the systemic circulation such as septicaemia or pulmonary infarction due to septic embolism. Sequelae of this kind have been observed, in similar cases, by Small and Turner (1947), and Cairns et al. (1947).

On the whole, septic thrombophlebitis of the major dural sinuses following penetrating injuries to the skull seems to be uncommon (Weber, 1957). Tönnis has encountered no case of thrombophlebitis resulting in cerebral abscess in his series of missile wounds up to 1941. In the 3 cases of Browder (1949) a compound fracture of the skull overlying the superior sagittal sinus was followed by fatal thrombophlebitis of the latter. The untoward event may cause rise in intracranial pressure and so contribute substantially to the fatal outcome. In missile wounds, phlebitis of a major dural sinus also has been observed at a distance from the brain wound and in the presence of primary healing of the scalp laceration. There is no satisfactory explanation as to the cause of this type of thrombosis (Cairns et al. 1947).

In our case infective material from a small-missile wound in the region of the glabella, after a considerable lapse of time, apparently had been carried within the superior longitudinal sinus in the direction of venous flow as far back as the torcular herophili, there giving rise to a septic phlebitis of the adjacent parts of the sagittal and right lateral sinuses; the latter anatomically represents, in the majority of cases, the direct continuation of the great sagittal sinus and from cases on record, appears to be the seat of preference of dural sinus thrombosis. Such discontinuity of spread would seem to be related to slowing-down of the blood flow within the confluens sinuum and the adjacent parts of the major dural sinuses draining into and from the confluent pool.

B. The convexity class

I. Penetrating head wounds associated with depressed fracture of the vault
(Peace time injuries)

There were 14 cases in the series, with 2 deaths. See Table 4.

1. Healing of scalp wound

A survey of the time interval between injury and operation in relation to the type of wound healing, whether per primary or secondary intention, reveals that no definite time limit can be demonstrated with regard to primary wound healing. Healing per primary union occurred after debridement carried out 11 and 12 days following injury, even in the presence of a discharging sinus as evidenced by cases 2.1.10 and 2.1.11. In case 2.1.14 the original scalp wound in the left frontal region was closed and already granulating when, six weeks after injury, the wound was re-opened and a frontal abscess evacuated. A soft rubber drain was removed after four days and did not interfere with primary healing of the wound.

On the other hand, there were two cases in which, despite early wound toilet on the first (case 2.1.1) and 4th day (case 2.1.5) respectively, the wound healing was per secondary union; in neither case primary wound closure was surgically attempted. Case 2.1.5 was a penetrating stab wound in a patient admitted on the 4th day after injury, and Proteus was cultured from the wound. Case 2.1.1 requires special comment. In this native girl of 14 the initial debridement which was carried out within a few hours after injury, was

Table 4. *Synopsis of penetrating head wounds associated with depressed fracture of the vault. (Peace time series)*

Case no.	Time of 1st surgical attempt	Operative findings and procedure	Wound healing	Special features
2.1.1	On admission	Depressed fracture left frontal, involving orbit and maxilla, not involving accessory sinuses; deep contusion left frontal lobe	per sec.	Incomplete debridement, intradural drainage. On 7th day brain exuding from gaping wound; re-suturing without drain. Convulsions; right facial weakness progressing to right hemiparesis and aphasia; patient drowsy and resistent. Purulent discharge from wound pockets, sequestrum removed (Fig. 30). Intercurrent miliary TBC. Recovered without gross neurological deficit. Keloid scar on forehead
2.1.2	within 24 hrs. of admission	Punctured wound left parietal, cluster of indriven bone chips; cleansing of track, 4 cm. deep; soft intracerebral drain for 2 days. Hemiplegia and aphasia	per pr.	Transient status epilepticus on 6th day; coliform bacilli isolated from brain wound. Left with hemiparesis
2.1.3	4 days	Stabwound left postero-parietal. Cleansing of track, dura closed, no drain	per pr.	Recovered. Coagulase-positive staphylococci isolated from brain wound
2.1.4	4 days	Deep cut wound right frontal (hit with an ax); debridement of brain wound, 8 cm. deep; 2 soft rubber drains	per pr.	Full recovery (Fig. 34). Bact. Coli isolated from brain wound
2.1.5	4 days	Penetrating stab wound left frontal; debridement, drain	per sec.	Recovered; Proteus isolated from wound
2.1.6	On admission	Depressed fracture, left temporo-parietal. Septic wound and discharging sinus. Pus and necrotic brain oozing through dura. Debridement. Intradural soft rubber drain, wound closure	per pr.	Slight weakness on right and aphasia, improved. Air encephalogram 3 weeks later: within normal. CSF. colourless, 2 lymphocytes
2.1.7	On admission	Penetrating stab wound left temporo-parietal; indriven bone chips; brain oozing. Cleansing of track from blood and pulped brain; ventricular tap; dura sealed off with muscle and fascia	Died on 5th day post op.	Necropsy: wound track extending into posterior horn of left ventricle; widespread meningitis and pyocephalus internus incl. 4th ventricle; traumatic cavity in left hemisphere; brain exuding through dura; subdural bleed in left middle fossa. No intracerebral clot, no brain abscess
2.1.8	Approx. one week	Osteitis and cortical abscess in left rolandic region	per sec.	Recovered with hemiparesis on right (Fig. 31)
2.1.9	9 days	Stabwound left frontal; discharging sinus; early type of brain abscess; soft rubber drain for 8 days	per sec.	Full recovery
2.1.10	11 days	Stab wound right parietal; osteitis and discharging sinus; hole in dura; excision and primary closure. No drain	per pr.	Recovery. (Jacksonian fits pre-operatively.)
2.1.11	12 days	Left frontal lobe abscess, local osteitis and discharging sinus; catheter drainage	per pr.	Recovery. Air encephalogram 14 days after operation showing slight shift to right
2.1.12	3 weeks	Left frontal, purulent discharging scalp wound, dura lacerated by bone spiculae, and adherent to brain; brain intact. Excision and closure without drain	per sec.	Subaponeurotic haematoma evacuated on 8th day; transient facial weakness on right. Recovered
2.1.13	4 weeks	Multiple injuries, two scalp lacerations left parietal, fissure in temporal squama; left hemiparesis (?)	per sec.	Protracted stupor and signs of brain stem damage. Bilateral occipital trephine openings in search for clot, ventriculography: no shift. Death 2 weeks afterward from purulent meningitis, abscess in right occipital lobe and pyocephalus internus

Table 4. (Continued)

Case no.	Time of 1st surgical attempt	Operative findings and procedure	Wound healing	Special features
2.1.14	6 weeks	On admission brain and CSF. oozing from scalp laceration in left frontal area; indriven bone chips. Wound granulating by the time of air encephalography which shewed a left frontal lobe abscess associated with intracerebral aerocele. Evacuation and soft rubber drain for 4 days	per pr.	Recovered without neurological sequelae

inadequate. Intradural drainage was instituted resulting in a dural leak. By the 7th day brain tissue was exuding between the stitches and required re-suturing of the wound, this time without drain. The patient had been on high doses of penicillin and sulphadiazine from

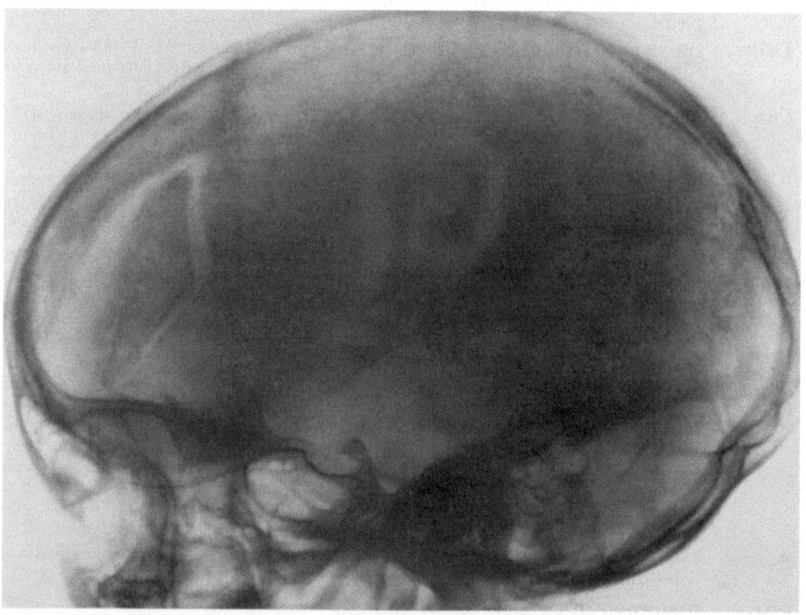

Fig. 30. Sequestra formation in a case of depressed fracture of the left frontal region with dura opened and contusion of the left frontal lobe. On admission, an incomplete debridement was carried out and intradural drainage installed. Dural leak required re-suturing on 7th day. Local osteitis developed and bony sequestra were removed. Achromobacter were cultured from the wound initially, later Esch. coli and staphylococci were isolated. Protracted wound healing. Pat. stayed in hospital for nearly 4 months (Case 2.1.1)

the onset; penicillin was replaced, after a fortnight, by streptomycin. Owing to deep frontal lobe damage, she was agitated and resistant, requiring unfailing watch and attention to the wound. From the 11th day, her hemiparesis improved while the wound was still discharging pus and debris. On several occasions bony sequestra were removed or delivered themselves from the wound (Fig. 30). She also had a series of epileptic convulsions. Despite an intercurrent miliary tuberculosis for which she was treated in an institution, she recovered eventually without disabling cerebral sequelae being left with a cicatricial keloid on the left forehead.

2. Complications

No instance of brain hernia was seen in this series, presumably owing to the principle of "closed box technique" in surgical repair being applied in most cases, together with chemotherapeutic control of infection. Drainage by means of soft rubber, also called Penrose drain, was used in the majority of cases, to serve as a channel to the intradural space for instillations of bactericidal solutions, and was removed after a few days; its function as an actual drain was considered of minor importance.

Case 2.1.8 illustrates the severe neurological deficit which may follow a cortical abscess, not even requiring drainage, if involving the rolandic region (Fig. 31). This patient is reminiscent of a case in BUCY's series (1938, case 6). His patient had a depressed fracture in the right central region overlying a small brain abscess from which several drops of thick pus were obtained; only the scalp wound was drained and the patient was left with a left-sided hemiplegia.

3. Involvement of the lateral ventricles

Head injuries penetrating the vault of the skull to involve the lateral ventricles are by far more common in missile wounds than in the field of civilian neurosurgery. Ventricular wounds associated with through-and-through bullet injuries may give rise to a primary or direct infection of the cerebrospinal fluid passages including the subarachnoid pools on the base of the brain. In the series under discussion ventricular involvement occurred thrice. The cases will be discussed now in brief.

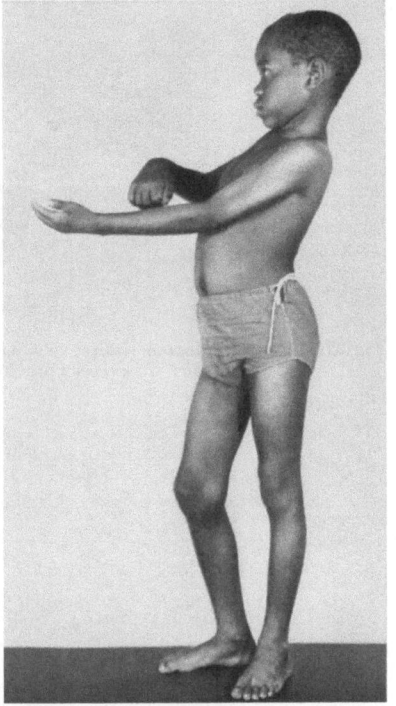

Fig. 31. To illustrate residual hemiparesis on right side, following cortical abscess in left rolandic region with local osteitis. Protracted course after superficial debridement, wound healing per sec. (Case 2.1.8)

Case 2.1.7. Stab wound in left temporo-parietal region with indriven bone. Debridement and primary closure on 4th day. Death 4 days later from meningitis and internal pyocephalus the cause of which was a communication of the wound track with the lateral ventricle not suspected during the wound toilet. (Most likely, this was a case of primary ventricular infection.)

This patient had sustained a penetrating stab wound to his left temporo-parietal region with superficially indriven bone chips, and was operated upon on the 4th day after injury when coagulated blood and pulped brain were cleansed out from the track. The wound was closed in two layers. The man died, rather unexpectedly, five days later i.e. nine days after wounding. Only at necropsy, it was realised that the brain wound had extended so far as to involve the posterior horn of the left lateral ventricle. No signs of suppuration were present to the naked eye, within the brain tissue. In marked contrast to this, there was a generalised meningitis involving the base as well as the convexity on either side of the midline, and a pyocephalus internus extending into the great cistern and the 4th ventricle. In addition, there was a subdural bleed on the floor of the left middle fossa, possibly related to a ventricular tap which had been carried out during debridement. The role of intracranial hypotension in penetrating head injuries has been discussed more fully in Chapter A (p. 32).

Case 2.1.13. Multiple scalp wounds healing up per granulationem. Protracted course with signs of brain stem involvement. Death following ventriculography. Necropsy revealed brain abscess in right occipital lobe and pyocephalus.

This man was admitted with multiple lacerations over the left parietal area as well as signs of brain stem involvement which failed to clear up during the ensuing four weeks. There was transient weakness of the left side. The scalp wounds were covered with fresh granulations when, in order to rule out a subdural clot, ventriculography was undertaken through bilateral occipital trephine openings well away from the granulating areas. No signs of an expanding mass were found on the X-rays. Five days after this procedure the patient developed signs of intracranial suppuration and despite full range chemotherapy, he succumbed from an abscess in the right occipital lobe associated with internal pyocephalus involving the entire ventricular system. Evidently, the infection here had been introduced with the ventricular cannula creeping along its track and giving rise, en route, to a brain abscess and eventually to ventricular suppuration. — More interesting is the following case.

Case 2.1.14. Depressed fracture of left frontal bone with dural laceration and cluster of indriven bone. Expectant treatment. 6 weeks later, a left frontal lobe abscess was evacuated successfully; it had formed around the dislodged bone and contained air which had entered the abscess cavity following an air encephalogram. No ventricular infection occurred and the wound healed p.pr. intention.

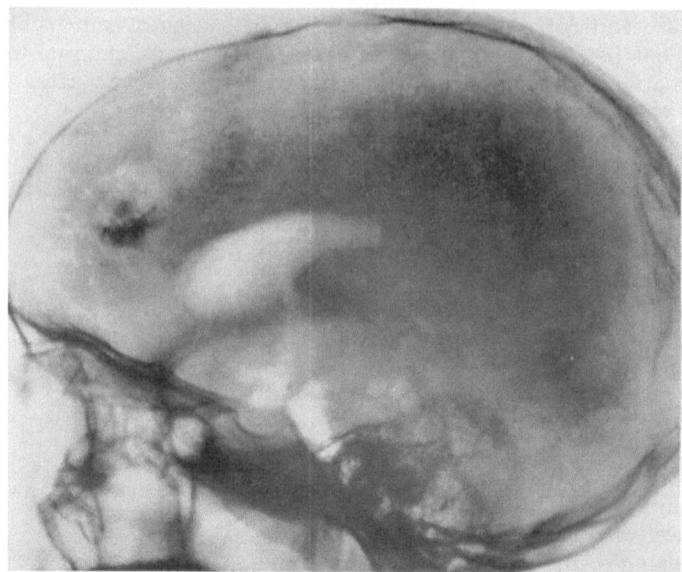

Fig. 32. Air encephalogram (lateral view with face up) in a case of left frontal lobe abscess following penetrating injury three weeks previously. Note indriven bone fragments. (Case 2.1.14)

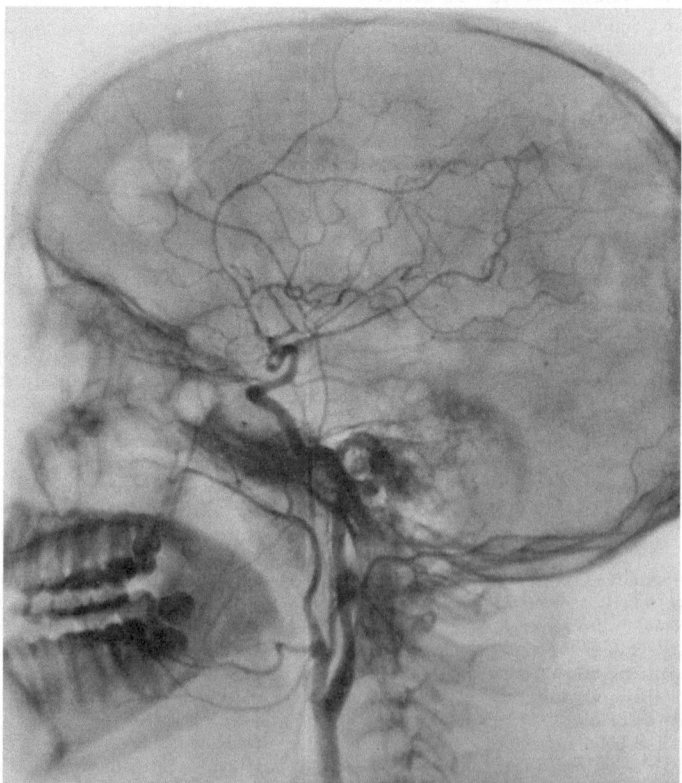

Fig. 33. Left carotid angiogram (lateral view) in the patient whose air encephalogram is shown in the preceding figure. Note displacement of the anterior cerebral group by the abscess in the left frontal lobe. The abscess cavity is visualized by air following air studies which were done 5 days prior to angiography. Patient recovered without neurological sequelae after evacuation of the abscess 6 weeks after injury. (Case 2.1.14)

This native boy, aged 18, was admitted to the King Edward VIII Hospital in Durban on September 29, 1958 with a depressed fracture of the left frontal squama, not involving the frontal sinus. Cerebrospinal fluid and semi-fluid brain were oozing from the wound. In the ward, the patient had a series of jacksonian fits which soon subsided. The X-rays showed a cluster of indriven bone fragments. Under conservative treatment the wound healed per granulationem. An air encephalogram on October 23, revealed a shift to the right (Fig. 32). Five days later, a left carotid angiogram was carried out and confirmed a left frontal abscess related to the retained bone chips. The significant finding on the angiogram, however, was a collection of air at the site of the abscess (Fig. 33). Apparently, the air had found its way, following air encephalography, from the ventricle into the cavity around the dislodged bone. The intracerebral aerocele was confirmed at the operation which was performed on November, 10, 1958, under general anaesthesia. On wedging out two loose bone pieces from within the brain, an abscess cavity, size of a peach, was opened up; it was filled with yellow pus which, during evacuation, became foaming, obviously due to admixture of air bubbles. The abscess had a well-defined, smooth pyogenic membrane that collapsed once its contents were washed out. The amount of pus was estimated to be approximately 15 ml. No cerebrospinal fluid leak occurred nor could a communication with the ventricle be disclosed during operation. A solution containing 20,000 units of penicillin was instilled into the abscess cavity through a Penrose drain which was removed after four days. The wound healed per primary union and the patient was discharged on 25 November, 1958, without neurological deficit and with a perfect, slightly depressed scar. — No follow-up notes were obtained from him after his discharge.

4. Bacteriology, chemotherapy

Relevant data will be seen from Table 5. The blanks indicate that no bacteriological examinations were carried out or the results are not available.

In the majority of cases routine chemotherapy viz. penicillin and sulpha drugs in various combinations, occasionally together with streptomycin, were given.

a) Effects on open scalp wound

In case 2.1.1 "open treatment" of an extensive and deep-reaching laceration of the scalp and brain was carried out. Seven days after injury, achromobacter (a potentially patho-

Table 5. *Bacteriology and chemotherapy (available data) in 14 cases of penetrating head wound and depressed fracture of the vault (Peace time series)*

Cace no.	Bacteriology	Chemotherapy	Outcome
2.1.1	Achromobacter initially; from 11th day on Esch. coli and coagulase-positive staphylococci	Penicillin and sulphadiazine; from 11th day onward penicillin replaced by streptomycin. (Period covered by chemotherapy = approx. 4 months)	Recovered; local osteitis and sequestra formation
2.1.2	*B. coli* (from brain)	chloromycetin	Primary healing
2.1.3	Coagulase-positive staphylococci (from debris)	Penicillin (20,000 u into brain wound)	Primary healing
2.1.4	*Esch.coli* (from drain in brain wound); foul smell	Penicillin topically; chloromycetin	Virtually primary healing (Fig. 34)
2.1.5	Proteus	Polymyxin (topical, intrathecal, intramuscular)	Recovered; healing per sec.
2.1.6		Penicillin-streptomycin	Primary healing
2.1.7		Penicillin-streptomycin from admission to death; chloromycetin (once)	Died from meningitis and pyocephalus, 9 days after injury
2.1.8	Local osteitis and cortical abscess		Per sec.
2.1.9	Pus from abscess cavity: staphyloc. albus et subtilis, not susceptible to current antibiotics	Penicillin, streptomycin, sulphatriad	Recovered; healing per sec.
2.1.10		Penicillin, sulphatriad topically	Healing per pr.
2.1.11			Healing per pr.
2.1.12			Recovered; healing per sec.
2.1.13		Penicillin from the onset, for 4 weeks; following ventriculography penicillin and streptomycin, and sulphadiazine	Died from brain abscess and *pyocephalus* 2 weeks after ventriculography in the presence of granulating wounds on head
2.1.14	(Aerogenous abscess in frontal lobe and granulating area on forehead.)	"Routine" chemotherapy before and after evacuation of abscess; 20,000 u penicillin into abscess cavity	Recovered. Wound healed per pr.

genic variety of schizomycetes) was isolated from the blood-mixed purulent discharge from the wound; the organisms proved to be sensitive to streptomycin and sulphonamides but not to penicillin; the latter subsequently was replaced by streptomycin while the administration of sulphadiazine was continued for 7 weeks. A protracted suppuration resulting in local osteitis and sequestra formation was possibly due to superinfection with E.coli and coagulase-positive staphylococci. There is but little doubt that this was facilitated by incomplete debridement and the presence of devitalized tissue outside and inside the dura mater with consequent gross delay in healing.

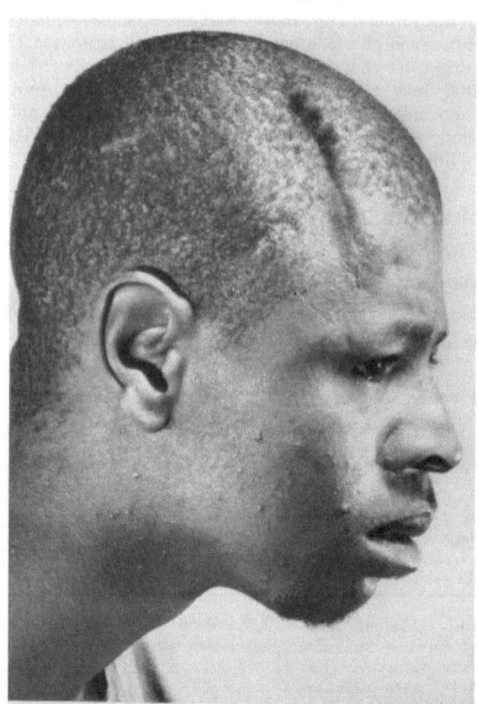

Fig. 34. To illustrate operative scar following primary wound healing in a patient who was hit with an ax and suffered a deep laceration of his right frontal lobe. Wound toilet was carried out 4 days after injury. Esch. coli were cultured from the brain wound and there was foul smell from it. Evacuation of a *subaponeurotic abscess* 11 days after operation did not interfere with wound healing. Chemotherapy locally and systematically (see table 5). Photo shows patient 7 weeks after operation. A suggestion of left facial weakness was the only neurological sequel. (Case 2.1.4)

As a rule, primary union of the scalp wound occurred in all cases where, after complete debridement, the wound was closed according to neurosurgical principles. Under appropriate chemotherapeutic "cover", bactericidal and bacteriostatic, primary healing was achieved even in the presence of septic wounds, localised osteitis of the vault, and a purulent discharging sinus after radical excision and closure; this is well exemplified by the cases 2.1.6, 2.1.10, and 2.1.11. In two instances, a subaponeurotic collection required incision on the 11th and 8th day respectively following operation without, however, interfering with wound healing.

In case 2.1.8 "open" treatment of a cortical abscess resulted in smouldering osteitis which, by the 5th week after the first surgical attack, resulted in a soft, atrophic scar.

b) Controlling intradural infection with E. coli and proteus

In addition to case 2.1.1 already mentioned, in two instances E. coli were isolated, on the 17th and 5th day respectively following primary wound toilet, from discharging Penrose drains which had been placed intradurally and issued through button holes. The depth of the brain wounds as measured from the surface was estimated 4 cm and 8 cm respectively in these two patients. In both, the infection responded satisfactorily to chloromycetin while the scalp lacerations healed up virtually per primary union. Additionally, in case 2.1.4 a subaponeurotic abscess, obviously communicating with the brain wound, was incised on the 11th day following primary closure, and pus from this abscess again yielded pure culture of E. coli. Fig. 34 illustrates the scar 4 weeks after operation. The patient returned for a check-up 7¹/₂ weeks after injury; he did very well then.

Case 2.1.5 presented with a stabwound and a sinus discharging thick pus from beneath the dura. *Proteus* vulgaris were isolated on culture. The infection responded dramatically to polymyxin which was administered into the brain wound through a rubber drain, as well as intrathecally and intramuscularly.

c) Early type of brain abscess

Purulent retention within the brain wound, so common in war injuries (which will be the subject of the following section) was encountered in this peace-time series only twice, viz. in case 2.1.1 already discussed, and in case 2.1.9 the history of which now follows.

Case 2.1.9. Early type of brain abscess in left frontal lobe following penetrating stab wound. Evacuation on 9th day of injury. Recovery.

This youngster, aged 19, received a stab wound to his left forehead and was admitted 8 days later with a discharging sinus. On admission, there was a tiny cut wound behind the left hair line surrounded by puffy, slightly elevated and fluctuent scalp. On pressure, copious sero-purulent discharge occurred from the wound. Except for a slight "ironing-out" of his right face there was no neurological or mental deviation. The optic discs were normal. X-rays showed a small roundish defect in the left frontal bone just in front of the coronal suture and about one inch to the left of the midline. One or two chips of bone were depressed but lodged near to the surface.

The following day, the 9th day after the injury, débridement was carried out under local anaesthesia. From a T-shaped incision the lesion was exposed. It was found that a small piece of the tabula interna had pierced through the dura. The opening was enlarged cross-like, while semi-liquid brain tissue and pus exuded from the hole in the dura. The brain surface lay close to the dura and no pulsation was visible. With the sucker an abscess cavity in the brain was entered the bottom of which was about 2 inches from the surface. More than $^{1}/_{2}$ oz. of purulent debris was removed from it by gentle suction, and the cavity then rinsed with saline solution and hydrogen peroxide. No haemostasis on the brain was needed. 20,000 units of penicillin were instilled into the abscess through a glove-drain which was secured to the skin. The skin edges were approximated by 5 silk stitches. Under systemic chemotherapy the patient made a quick recovery. The drain was removed after 8 days. There was but little discharge from the wound which healed up per granulationem. The patient was restored to full working capacity within 4 weeks of the operation.

Comment. In this case bacteriology from a brain abscess which was evacuated on the 9th day following a penetrating wound, yielded skin saprophytes only, not susceptible to chemotherapeutic agents in common use, and possibly not even pathogenic. Since bacteriological examination was not repeated after the operation we do not know whether super-infection occurred after surgical exposure and drainage. If so, it was kept well under control by post-operative chemotherapy. Although the wound healing was secondary, there was no problem of protracted drainage, separation of the stitches or brain herniation in this case nor in any other in the series under consideration.

d) Purulent ventriculitis and pyocephalus internus

Once the infection has reached the lateral ventricle be it via the original brain wound or due to rupture of a brain abscess into the ventricle, pyocephalus internus and externus will ensue almost inevitably. Suppuration within the 3rd ventricle is liable to produce devastating effects on the hypothalamic structures with the well-known sequelae regarding autonomous and endocrine control. In addition, accumulation of large amounts of pus within the ventricular cavities and the greater cisterns in the middle and posterior fossae, is likely to be followed by one or the other type of coning. It is thus natural that pyocephalus is usually a terminal stage offering poor prognosis. In WEBER's series (1957) of 73 brain abscesses only one single case of pyocephalus is mentioned. It followed rupture of a deep-seated frontal abscess into the left lateral ventricle. The patient succumbed within 3 days despite repeated penicillin instillations into the ventricle. — GURDJIAN and WEBSTER, in 1948, reported survival in one of their cases.

Symptomatology and surgical management of brain abscess rupturing into the ventricle was reviewed lately by GUND[1] who had two patients under his care. From the abstract of his paper it would appear that neither excision nor open drainage and chemotherapy can offer much hope for these patients.

This is also borne out in a paper by BALLANTINE and SHEALY. In their series of 44 brain abscesses there were 15 fatalities and, among these, 14 were due to either rupturing of the abscess into the ventricle or brain stem displacement at the tentorial or tonsillar levels.

Thus surgical management must aim at early diagnosis of brain abscess in order to prevent ventricular rupture rather than to treat this complication; however, few would go as far as BALLANTINE and SHEALY who advocate emergency surgery as a routine measure soon a brain abscess is diagnosed.

---

[1] GUND, A.: Ist die Behandlung eines ins Liquorsystem eingebrochenen Hirnabscesses aussichtsreich ? Acta neurochir. **7**, 446 (1959).

Table 6. *Survey (available data) of 12 selected cases of early type of brain abscess following penetrating missile wound (war injuries)*

Case no.	Time of follow-up débridement after wounding	Findings in loco	Postoperative course
2.2.1	unknown	Early abscess left parietal, quadrangular scalp defect; numerous retained bone chips. Drainage of abscess; sulphonamide powder into abscess	Persistent hemiparesis, hemianopia, and aphasia, high temperature; big herniation controlled by lumbar taps which open up a deep track the walls of which pulsate and granulate 14 days after operation. — Died with persistent cerebral fungus and gross hemispherical oedema; narrow track without retention, en route to enlarged lateral ventricle
2.2.2	22 days	Early abscess right parietal beneath entrance wound obstructed by bone fragments. Debridement and tight drainage	Healing per granulationem
2.2.3	18 days	Right frontal abscess beneath huge infected cerebral fungus and extensive scalp loss (had been 5 times operated on previously). Debridement and drain	Repeated lumbar taps to control herniation, sudden meningitis after 7 days; 10 ml. of fluid aspirated from contralateral ventricle. Died 9 days after drainage. Necropsy (Prof. R. Rössle): purulent meningitis in both middle fossae and right anterior fossa; unsuspected fresh abscess in right temporal lobe
2.2.4	12 days	Left frontal abscess beneath patent entrance wound (see Fig. 35). Drainage	Alternating herniation and recession, drain pushed out by fungating brain; frontal lobe syndrome. Died 5 days after drainage. Firm dural barrier surrounding abscess (Fig. 36). Abscess ruptured into ventricle, gross hemispherical oedema
2.2.5	20 days	Early abscess left parietal, removal of numerous bone fragments; drain	Aphasia; no herniation developed; 5 days after op. foul smell from the wound; a fortnight thereafter abscess cavity with pulsating walls covered with granulations. 1 year after wounding solid scar, sunk and fixed to underlying structures; right hemiplegia; no fits
2.2.6	18 days	Entry wound right frontal, obstructed by depressed fragments; sinus on scalp with pulsating purulent discharge; abscess size of walnut opened up by lumbar tap; debridement and sulphonamide powder, drain	Discharge from wound with foul smell; herniation alternating with deep recession associated with bradycardia, vomiting and headache; normal temperature. Lumbar fluid remained clear: patient euphoric. Wound healed per granulat. Solid indrawn scar 8 weeks after wounding
2.2.7	15 days	Left frontal early abscess; opened up and soft rubber drain inserted. (Brain had been oozing from wound and fungus developed 5 days after wounding; fungus receded after lumbar tap but returned within 24 hours)	Aphasia, right facial weakness and paresis of right arm. Drain recovered 6 weeks after operation, from a granulating cavity, 1 inch deep. Wound closed 10 weeks after operation. See Fig. 41
2.2.8	26 days	Huge infected brain hernia and considerable skin loss in right parietal area, see Fig. 42. Octopus drain	Died 5½ weeks after debridement, with parkinsonian symptoms. Necropsy: Shallow abscess cavity covered with granulations and occupying the greater part of right hemisphere, extending close to basal ganglia; focus of encephalitis posteriorly; no ventricular involvement, no meningitis
2.2.9	unknown	Right frontal abscess behind infected cerebral fungus, considerable scalp loss. Drainage	Died within 7 weeks from drainage
2.2.10	unknown	Left fronto-parietal early abscess behind pocketed and infected cerebral fungus; considerable scalp loss. X-rays show deeply indriven bone fragments; 16 of these were removed during debridement	Died within 8 weeks; postmortem specimen see Fig. 43

Table 6 (Continued)

Case no.	Time of follow-up débridement after wounding	Findings in loco	Postoperative course
2.2.11	unknown	Purulent retention within deep pocket opened up by lumbar tap, above right ear, see Fig. 37. Despite relaxation incision primary wound closure failed. Drainage	Followed up for 4 weeks only. Discharged with small defect in scalp and a wound crater covered with healthy-looking granulations
2.2.12	10 days	Tangential missile wound in right parietal area with indriven bone, first debrided 2 days after wounding, gauze plug inserted. Subcutaneous cerebral fungus developed and became infected; secondary debridement and drainage	Healing per granulationem

In the above series both patients with pyocephalus internus died, and they were the only deaths in this series. In both patients the pyocephalus was an unsuspected finding on the post mortem table. One patient (case 2.1.7) had a 9 days' treatment with penicillin and di-hydrostreptomycin systemically; the same agents, together with sulphadiazine, were administered in case 2.1.13 for a period of 6 weeks.

The two cases may serve to illustrate the difficulties in diagnosis and treatment, surgical and by chemotherapy, to be faced in such instances. Ventricular involvement may be not obvious even during operation and cleansing of a brain wound, especially in the presence of a narrow track as it is common in stab wounds.

II. The early type of brain abscess (frühabscess) following penetrating missile wounds (war injuries)

In marked contrast to peace-time injuries which were the subject of the preceding section, the early type of brain abscess or *Frühabscess* is common in missile wounds under the conditions of war.

During the war 1939—1945 the management of the early brain abscess was subject to much controversy and one can hardly say that general agreement has been reached as to the most suitable method of treatment to be applied under the prevailing circumstances. The controversy went on after the war in the light of new developments in chemotherapy and of practical experiences gained during the Korea crisis.

In Table 6 are listed 12 cases of early brain abscess treated in 1941 at the neuro-surgical unit of the Charité in Berlin, together with their relevant features, clinical and post mortem, as derived from data available to the author. These cases were selected from a much larger series treated at the same unit. The selection was made with a view to certain physio-pathological aspects brought out by a close study of these selected cases which, in this respect, represent the whole series. The cases summarized in Table 6, however, are not representative regarding the late results obtained which is obvious from the fact that among the 12 cases listed there were 6 deaths. The over-all mortality rate is reflected by such figures as given by PEIPER who reported 17% deaths among 583 infected cranio-cerebral wounds due to missiles, and those by TÖNNIS whose mortality was 32,3% in 915 open brain injuries[1].

1. Definition of early brain abscess

The so-called "Frühabscess" is equivalent to "acute pyogenic abscess", a term used by CAIRNS and assoc. (1947), viz. purulent retention within a brain wound or a missile track occurring at a time while the scalp wound is still in the process of healing per granulationem (SPATZ, 1941; footnote on p. 197, and Fig. 12a on page 185).

---

[1] Data derived from: SCHALTENBRAND, G.: Naturforschung und Medizin in Deutschland 1939—1946 (Fiat Review of German Science) Band 81, Neurologie, Teil II, p. 139. Wiesbaden: Dieterich'sche Verlagsbuchhandlung.

Consequently, the patients suffering from an early brain abscess present either with a suppurating wound or wounds of the scalp or with a sinus discharging frank pus (Fig. 35). The discharge may clearly show pulsation. In the average case, the contents of the brain wound or track become gradually purulent during and by the end of the second week after wounding (TÖNNIS, 1941). A similar sequence of events has been found in experimental animals (IRSIGLER and SÜDHOF, 1943). By this time also some sort of demarcation of the abscess by a pyogenic membrane has been reached, and, on the surface of the brain, the

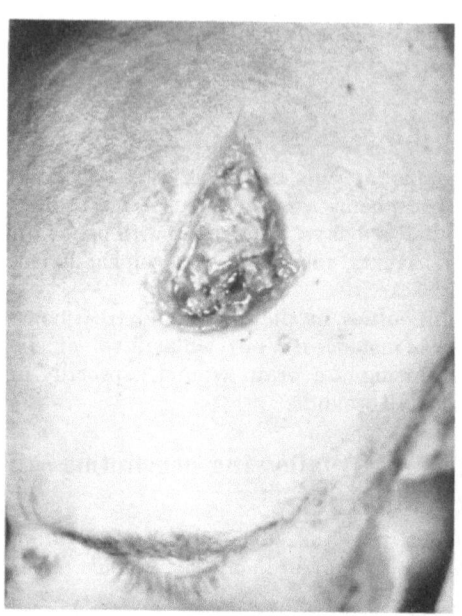 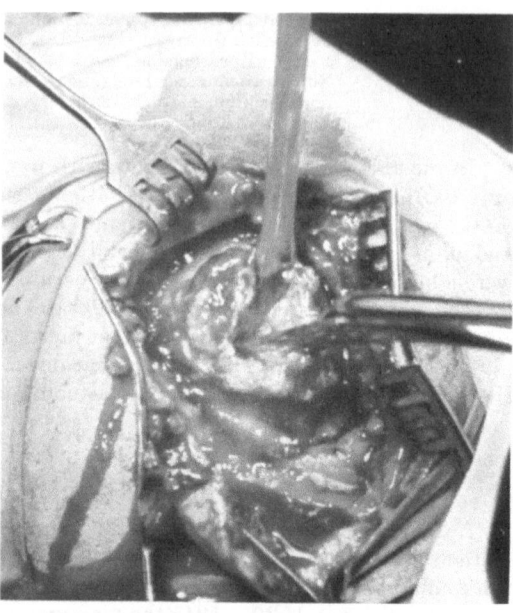

a   b

Fig. 35. a Early brain abscess in left frontal lobe due to missile injury. Appearance of wound 12 days after initial debridement and excision of scalp. The wound had been plugged with gauze and no attempt at primary wound closure had been made. — Note bruises on dorsum of nose indicating cranio-facial injury. b The abscess being opened and emptied by means of sucker and grasping forceps. Note thick capsule which has formed by the 12th day. — The man died 5 days after drainage of the abscess from sudden haemorrhage from the internal maxillary and lingual arteries. See following figure (Case 2.2.4)

entry into the abscess appears well circumwalled by meningo-cortical adhesions around the periphery (Fig. 36) which are tough enough to prevent spread of infection on to the convexity of the brain unless this protective barrier is disrupted by careless handling.

2. Failure of initial surgery

The first surgical approach to an open brain wound must aim at complete and final closure, if necessary by means of plastic procedures (Fig. 26). Failure to achieve primary closure or inadequacy of first surgical attack will almost inevitably result in persistence or recurrence of an open wound (due to separation of stitches) bound to develop infection of the pericranium and bone, and facilitating bacterial invasion into deep structures with a whole gamut of intradural suppurations including cerebral thrombophlebitis and ventricular rupture with purulent ventriculitis and pyocephalus (case 2.2.4).

Failure to restore the physiological "closed box mechanism" will, in addition, result in pressure fluctuations, often abrupt and precipitous, and give rise to cerebral fungus obstructing, temporarily or persistently, the bone defect in the vault, and alternating with low pressure states. The latter have been observed either spontaneously (TÖNNIS) and

Fig. 36. Necrospy specimen of patient shown in foregoing Fig. 35. Early type of frontal lobe abscess 17 days after wounding. Note firm meningeal adhesions around entry to abscess, and oedema of ipsilateral hemisphere. On the cut surface of this specimen it was found that the abscess had ruptured into the lateral ventricle giving rise to purulent ventriculitis and basal meningitis (Case 2.2.4)

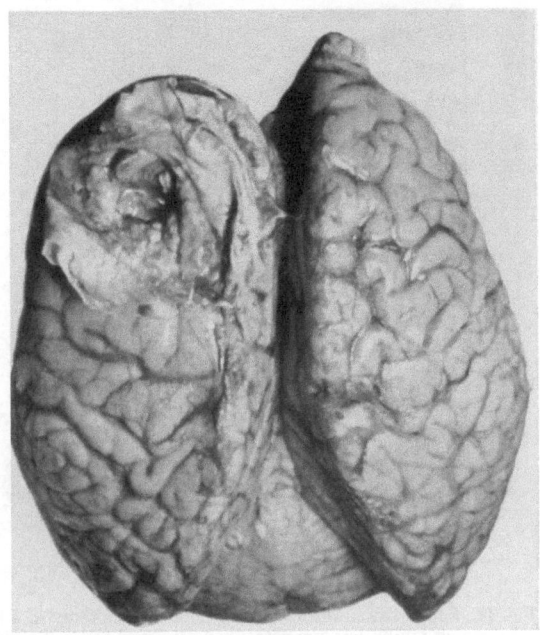

without apparent cerebrospinal fluid leak or, more often, following repeated lumbar taps to promote reduction (recession) of the brain hernia as illustrated in Fig. 37. Finally, those who survive will be left either with intracerebral smooth-walled cysts, often multilocular and connected with the ventricle (SPATZ, 1941) as shown in Fig. 38 or with dense fibrous scarring with its inherent tendency to shrinkage, involving all layers from the skin to the ependyma of the lateral ventricle. This kind of scar, being an important epileptogenic focus, as recognized long ago by FOERSTER and PENFIELD, often necessitates surgical excision years after injury (Fig. 39). Jacksonian fits may result from circumscribed, delicate meningo-cerebral adhesions (Fig. 40). CAIRNS has stated that incidence of epilepsy after cerebral fungus amounts to almost 100%.

3. Intracranial hypotension

TÖNNIS (1941) has drawn attention to episodes of low pressure occurring in cases of early pyogenic abscess, especially following repeated lumbar taps. Instead of a fungating mass, one is surprised to find a deep recession or crater exposing the bottom of the abscess cavity which, by this time, usually is formed by a granulating membrane. Episodic hypotension may occur also without apparent cause, preceded and again followed by raised pressure as evinced by cerebral herniation. This is well exemplified by case 1.3 in Chapter A (p. 54); this patient with a missile wound through the frontal sinus had been re-explored 20 days after wounding. Six days following

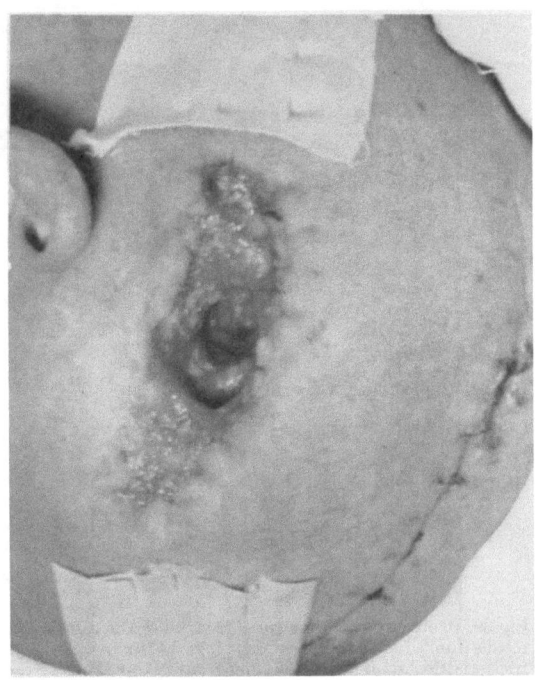

Fig. 37. To illustrate deep recession of brain beneath dura mater following lumbar tap in a case of early brain abscess due to missile wound above right ear. Appearance of wound nine days after tight drainage. Note granulating area occupying original wound, and fresh scar in parietal region resulting from relaxation incision

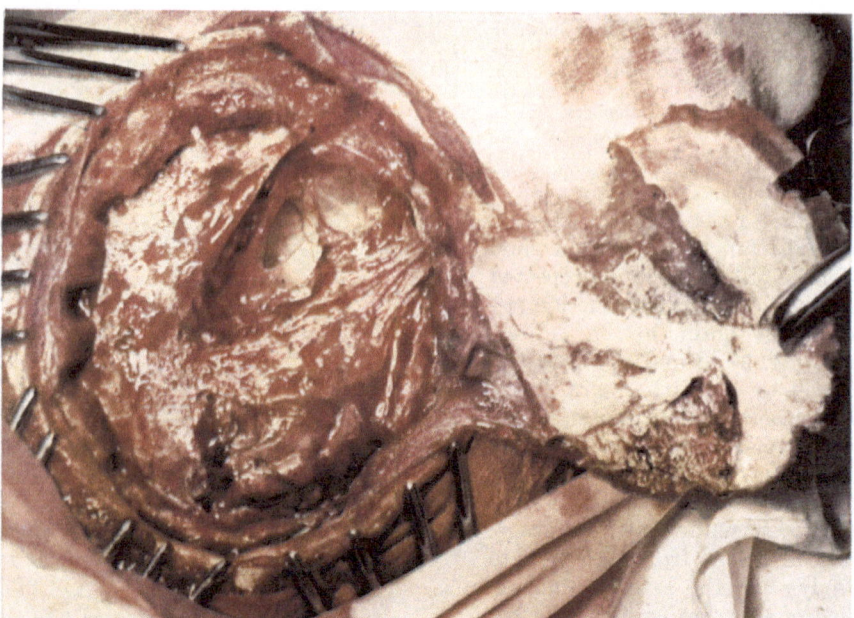

Fig. 38. Photo taken during right frontal craniotomy in a boy, aged 15, who, at the age of 7, had suffered a car accident which left him with a comminuted fracture of the right side of the vault of his skull and left spastic hemiplegia. There was gross atrophy of his left arm and hand. No operation had been performed at the time of injury. Jacksonian fits developed with an adversive aura. Air studies revealed atrophic type of hydrocephaly and a multiloculated intracerebral cyst beneath the fractured vault communicating with the right lateral ventricle. Note absence of a solid scar so common in infected brain wounds. Through defect in the dura mater and the roof of the cyst replacing the greater part of the right frontal lobe, the ependyma of the enlarged frontal horn can be seen. — The roof of the cyst was excised and the dural defect closed with a fascial graft. The sylvian group was embedded in, and constricted by, dense fibrous tissue; obviously, this had caused permanent hemiplegia

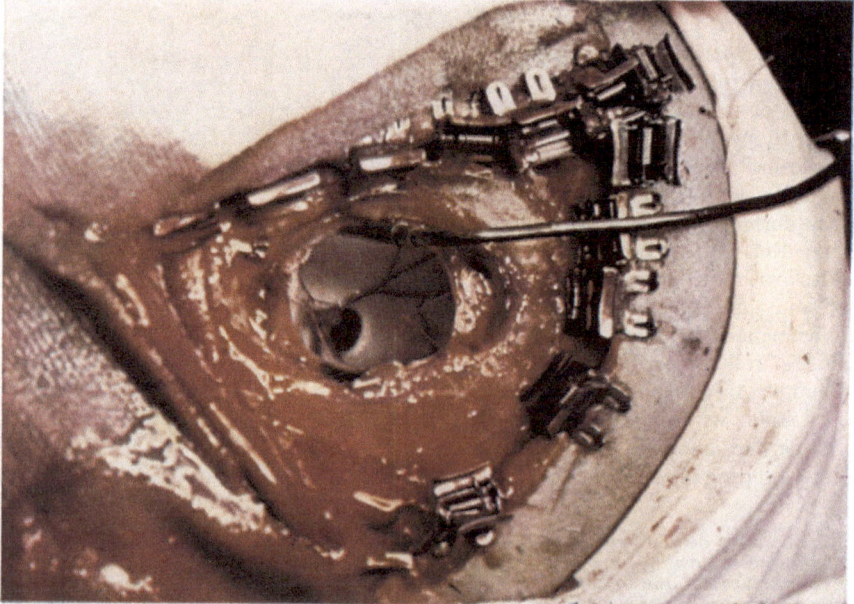

Fig. 39. Photo taken during craniotomy over the right frontal region. A cranio-cerebral scar following penetrating missile injury has been excised in toto right down to the dilated lateral ventricle. Note ependymal lining of ventricle and foramen of MONRO which is dilated allowing view into 3rd ventricle. A small electric light attached to a pliable rod has been introduced into the ventricle (1941)

Fig. 40. Photo taken during craniotomy under local anaesthesia. Dura mater incised and reflected to expose circumscribed meningo-cerebral adhesion due to penetrating injury. The patient, a man of 23, was suffering from jacksonian fits merging, at times, into a status epilepticus. Pulling during exposure and excision of this meningo-cortical scar produced an epileptic attack. Air encephalography in this case had disclosed a significant lack of subarachnoid air over the convexity involved (1941)

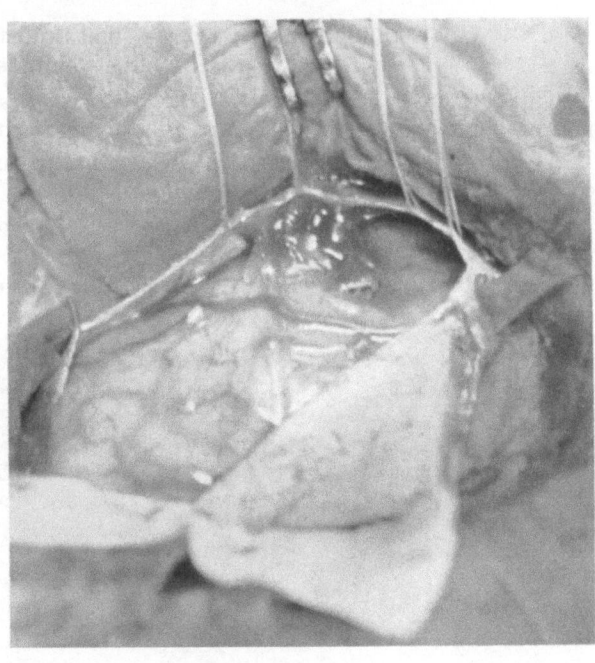

operation and drainage when re-dressing the wound, a deep recess was found to have replaced the fungus of the previous day, and followed anew by herniation next day. There was no cerebrospinal fluid leakage nor any communication with the ventricle. During the stage of low pressure there was no striking change in the patient's condition, his pulse rate being 72 and temperature 37° C. Colloidal solutions as well as normal saline were administered in an effort to replenish the body fluids.

Lumbar or cisternal taps, repeatedly and judiciously carried out are a convenient and often recommended method to promote reduction of a cerebral fungus and "opening up" a deep abscess cavity or track as illustrated in Fig. 37 unless a too narrow opening in the cranial vault precludes the fungus from receding; the result is a kind of incarceration. Longstanding cerebral fungi may acquire increased consistency and become firmly attached to the pericranium. Obviously, reduction of such chronic herniations by with-drawal of lumbar or cisternal fluid becomes impracticable.

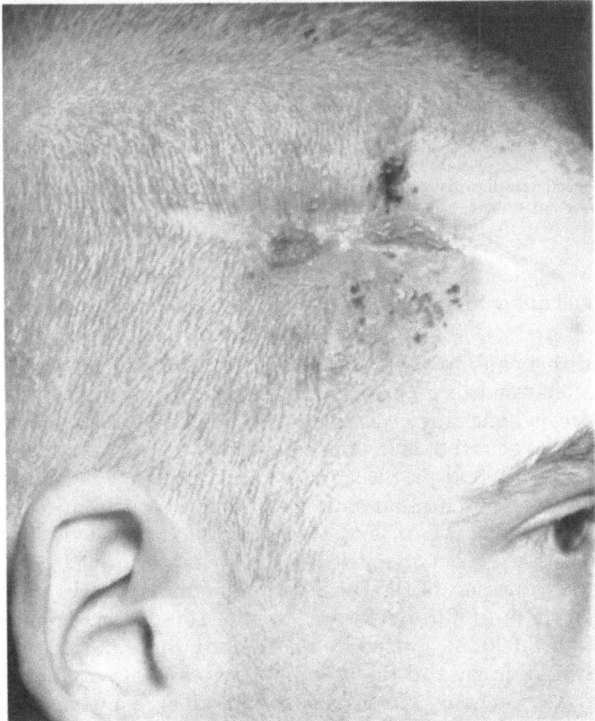

Fig. 41. To show scar following early brain abscess in left frontal region due to missile wound. On the 5th day after wounding pulped brain had been oozing from the wound. A brain hernia developed together with a right hemiparesis and aphasia. 15 days after wounding the abscess was drained. Alternating episodes of herniation and recession followed. Three weeks after operation 3 fluid ounces of thick pus were removed from the cavity by suction. The wound healed within 10 weeks of drainage of the abscess. The patient recovered from his disabling neurological symptoms (Case 2.2.7). Note that right and left sides are reversed in this picture

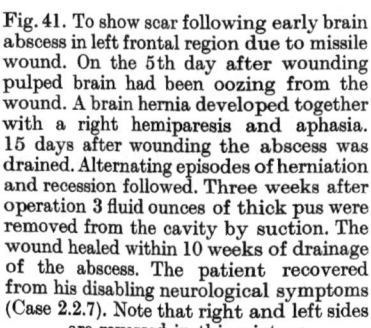

4. Accumulation of cerebro-spinal fluid within the surface pools.
(So-called hydrocephalus externus.)

This is found to be a characteristic feature persisting through the entire phase of pressure fluctuations which accompany open treatment of the early type of brain abscess.

That we are dealing here with an external rather than an internal type of hydrocephalus appears obvious from the following:

1. *Ventricular taps yielding negligible or small amounts of fluid and therefore failing to provide relief of pressure.*

This is exemplified by the two case histories (Table 6) which follow:

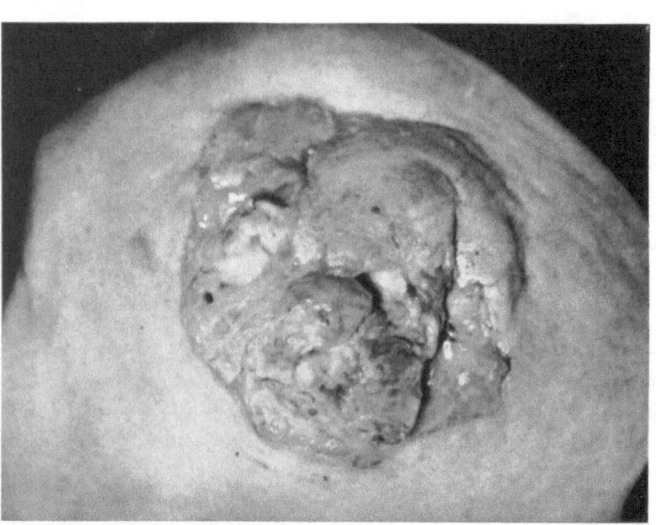

Fig. 42. Cauliflower-like fungation following penetrating missile wound and shattering of the vault of skull on the right. Several surgical attempts had been made before this man reached the neurosurgical unit, 26 days after wounding as shown above. Staphylococci were isolated from the lumbar fluid. Despite radical debridement and drainage of several deep-seated abscesses the patient succumbed eventually with symptoms of basal ganglia involvement as described in text, at a stage when the bottom of the abscesses had reached skin level and was covered with healthy-looking granulations. (Case 2.2.8)

a) *Case 2.2.7.* This was a man with a left frontal abscess debrided 15 days after wounding. Progressive right hemiparesis was noted two weeks following debridement. A lumbar tap at this time yielded 40 ml. of clear fluid opening up the abscess cavity. There was no purulent retention within the abscess; subsequently the right arm became paralysed. When, on the following day, both posterior horns were tapped with a brain cannula they were found to harbour a few ml. of clear fluid. Air insufflation into the ventricles revealed a marked shift. Again herniation developed and 3 days following ventriculography 60 ml. were withdrawn by the lumbar route. From the abscess now approximately 3 fluid ounces of thick pus were removed by suction, and tight octopus drainage installed. The patient recovered eventually including his hemiplegia. Fig. 41 shows the scar 10 weeks after operation.

b) *Case 2.2.8.* A soldier, aged 30, with a right parietal missile wound was admitted with a cauliflower-like encephalitic fungation of considerable size, and re-explored 26 days after wounding (Fig. 42). The vault was found to be shattered and heavily infected, indriven bone chips were removed, and an abscess, about 4 in. deep and eccentrically situated, was evacuated and drained with two *octopus* rubber tubes. The patient received 380 ml. of fresh blood and was put on heavy dosage of sulphonamides (eleudron). Two days later a few ml. of lumbar fluid were withdrawn from which staphylococci were cultured. The patient was again hydrated with blood, polyvinylpyrrolidon and concentrated glucose. The same day a ventricular tap was performed and 3 or 4 ml. were removed from the left posterior horn. During the ensuing 4 weeks daily lumbar taps were performed and amounts of fluid between 80 and 150 ml. were removed on each occasion totaling more than 2,000 ml. gained by the lumbar route during this period while the fungus gradually settled down and the bottom of two abscess cavities, covered by healthy-looking granulations reached skin level. Wound closure by means of a rotating flap was considered.

However, the patient developed a parkinsonian picture with pyrexia and died $5^1/_2$ weeks after debridement i.e. $9^1/_2$ weeks after wounding. Post mortem examination revealed a huge granulating area reinforced by a pyogenic membrane 3 mm. thick, occupying the greater part of the right hemisphere, and extending into close vicinity of the basal ganglia. There was an area of localised cerebritis posteriorly but no meningitis and no communication with the ventricle were apparent to the naked eye. *No internal hydrocephalus was present.*

2. *Post mortem specimens exhibiting* no ventricular enlargement or a mild degree of dilatation only which is out of proportion with regard to the amounts of fluid gained by the lumbar route.

This will become clear from Figs. 43—45 and their respective subscripts.

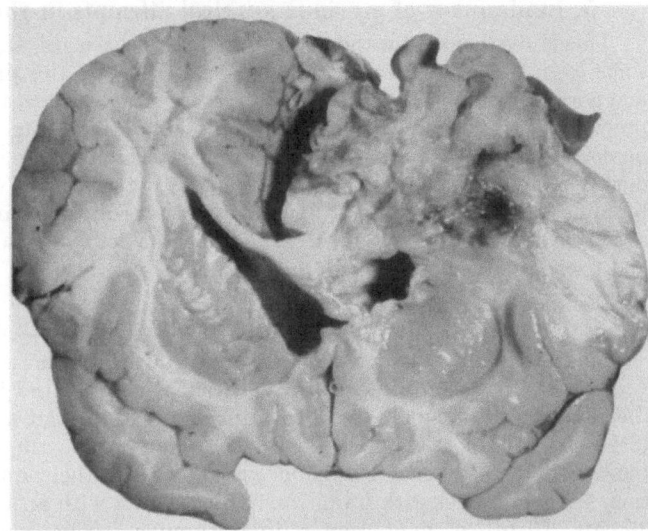

Fig. 43

Fig. 43. Post mortem specimen (coronal view). Tangential missile wound in right rolandic and parietal areas. Patient admitted with fungating cerebritis; 16 retained bone chips were removed. Death occurred 56 days after operation. Shift of the midline to side of continued herniation. Moderate enlargement of contralateral ventricle

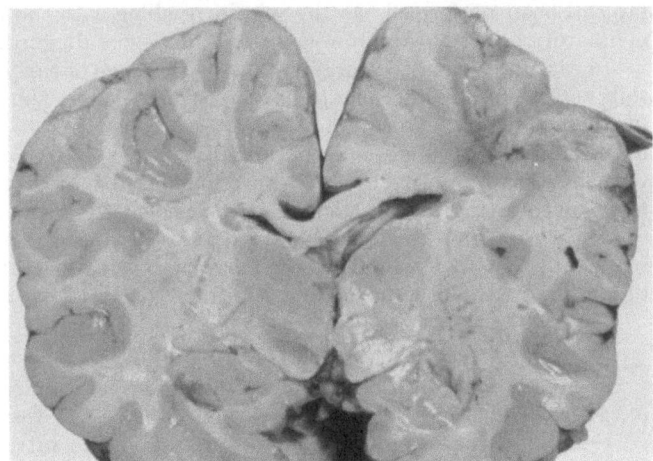

Fig. 44

Fig. 44. Post mortem specimen (coronal view). Condition following debridement and tight drainage of early type of brain abscess. No residual abscess. Shrinkage of hemisphere involved. Slight enlargement of the ipsilateral ventricle

Fig. 45. Early brain abscess following missile wound. Condition 12 days after wounding. Negligible enlargement oft left trigonum. Note absence of elevation of roof of lateral ventricle beneath a left parasagittal abscess

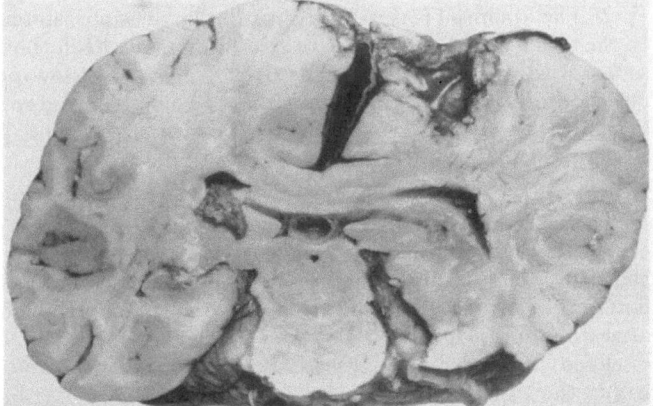

Fig. 45

5. Inadequacy of previous surgical attempts in the cases under discussion

This is evidenced by the presence, in every case, of an infected wound or discharging sinus over the cranial vault and, in some cases, by the presence of a large area of scalp and pericranial loss. This, surely, increased in extent with the number of surgical attempts previously made, most of them in the forward area (Fig. 42). In many of the wounded numerous retained bone chips, often of considerable size, had to be removed during re-debridement of the abscess (Fig. 46). Except in those cases with an entry wound obstructed by bone fragments, a fungating mass was present as a rule, and since no penicillin was available at that time (1941—1942) sulphonamides were used, rather generously, by mouth and topically by frosting with sulphonamide powder (Fig. 27).

6. Moderate degree of ventricular dilatation

This has been recounted and exemplified by clinical as well as post mortem experiences. In none of the cases in the group ventricular tap resulted in substantial relief of pressure, the amount of fluid obtained ranging between nil and a few ml., on the whole tending to be slightly more pronounced on the side opposite the abscess (Fig. 43). Needling for the ventricles may even be unsuccessful owing to their smallness, displacement or distortion. We never met with frank pus. In case 2.2.3 with an unsuspected right temporal lobe abscess, 10 ml. of fluid were gained through the brain cannula from the left ventricle 2 days before death. In case 2.2.4 (Fig. 36) who died from pyocephalus no ventricular tap had been performed. On the whole, needling with the brain cannula was of little avail and hardly contributory from the point of view of diagnosis.

In case 2.2.7 ventriculography during the stage of early abscess revealed a considerable shift across the midline. The patient recovered during the ensuing 10 weeks after debridement (Fig. 41). No indication of an abscess in addition to the one debrided, was obtained during the entire course of convalescence. No explanation can be offered as to the cause of such shift; however, it should be remembered that cerebral thrombophlebitis has been found accounting for ventricular displacement by PENNYBACKER (1945). It seems reasonable to assume that major fluctuations of pressure as evidenced by fungation and recession (Fig. 37) are associated with some degree of transient ventricular displacement to the one or the other side (Fig. 43), more likely to the side of the cerebral hernia.

7. Concluding remarks

Although there are obvious limitations some conclusions may be drawn from the foregoing discussion. They can be summarized as follows:

1. Changes often precipitous and alternating, in intracranial pressure which characterise the stage of "open" treatment of early brain abscess, evidently are hydrodynamic in nature and closely related to the absorption rather than production of cerebrospinal fluid.

2. The essential feature is accumulation of cerebrospinal fluid within the external pools on the surface and at the base of the brain, not within the ventricles as generally assumed so far. Also, lack of clinical signs during episodes of low pressure, as indicated by sudden recession of a previous fungating mass, would seem more consistent with changes in the amount of "external" fluid than changes in size of, and pressure within, the ventricular system.

8. Early fatalities

There are two in our series. Case 2.2.4 died 5 days after debridement which was carried out 12 days after wounding. Necropsy disclosed rupture of the abscess into the lateral ventricle with ensuing suppurative ventriculitis and purulent collection in the great cistern. In case 2.2.3 who had been operated on for a right fronto-temporal abscess 18 days after wounding, and succumbed 9 days after the operation necropsy by Professor R. RÖSSLE disclosed purulent meningitis in both middle fossae and an unsuspected fresh abscess within the right temporal lobe.

Case 2.2.4 was the only one with frank burst of an early abscess into the lateral ventricle. Case 2.2.3 was the only one in which an abscess (in the temporal lobe) was missed while an abscess in the frontal lobe had been drained.

There was no subdural abscess in the group under discussion.

9. Late fatalities

Four patients died at a late stage, roughly speaking between 8 and 16 weeks following operation. No detailed reports on necropsy findings have been obtained in these cases. Post mortem specimens of two patients are shown in Figs. 36 and 43. In case 2.2.8 a localised area of encephalitis adjoining the pyogenic membrane of a huge abscess was found but no frank pus was present within the ventricles nor in the great cistern. However, insidious ventricular infection must possibly be admitted (though confirmed under the microscope only) in this as well as the other cases with fatal outcome.

Increasing *dehydration* is likely to become apparent clinically in patients with a protracted course. Obviously, actual fluid loss through frequent lumbar taps is only one of the factors contributing to this condition which gradually merges into emaciation and marasmus. Thus, early and persistent control of dehydration is imperative. In the above series, repeated transfusions of fresh blood as well as infusions of colloidal (macromolecular) solutions or of concentrated plasma have been found of great assistance albeit not effective in all such cases; the mixture we used most often if blood was not available, was vinyl-pyrrolidon or collidon (periston). Eventually, with the abscess and its perifocal reaction approaching the deep structures near the midline, a parkinsonian syndrome with rigidity, tremor (at rest and on intention) with attendant autonomic responses such as profuse sweating and other signs of lost temperature control, may develop and forecast approaching disaster. We were sometimes struck by the contrast between the rapidly and irrevocably declining clinical course and the local appearance of a well-developed pyogenic membrane carpeted with healthy-looking granulations and approaching the skin level.

10. Critical remarks regarding ipsilateral ventricular dilatation

Localised dilatation involving the ipsilateral ventricle in debrided brain wounds has been evidenced, by encephalography, as early as the 2nd week after injury (Fig. 46). It evidently indicates and replaces circumscribed loss of cerebral tissue. As pointed out by TÖNNIS (1941) it can not be interpreted as being due, at such an early stage, to a contracting scar as formerly assumed. It should be clear that this type of ventricular enlargement, giving the impression of a diverticulum or recess in broad communication with the ventricle, is different from the cleft-like extension or elongation of the lateral angle of the lateral ventricle occasionally seen in excessive cerebral fungation with or without an underlying abscess. The ipsilateral ventricle may be displaced as a whole en route to the outlet in the cranial vault plugged by the fungating mass (SPATZ, 1941). It is this state of affairs which has been feared and found, as early as 20 days after wounding, by WEBSTER et al. (1946ᵃ) and others at operations on early abscess following penetrating missile wounds. It has not been encountered in the present series although well demonstrated in animal experiments by the author (IRSIGLER, 1942); a characteristic feature is the excentrically placed wound track within the fungus (Fig. 47).

O'CONNELL (1943, 1948) has advocated a diverticulum-like dilatation of the lateral ventricle forming the centre of a cerebral fungus and causing progressive fungation; this seems somewhat hypothetical and has not been confirmed in any of our cases in which cerebral herniation was persistently held under control by lumbar or cisternal taps to the effect that deep recession was a frequent occurrence; it is possibly significant that such recession was more often encountered in those who survived.

With the bottom of the abscess cavity approaching the skin level the roof of the lateral ventricle comes nearer to the surface (RIECHERT, 1942) and ventricular rupture may well

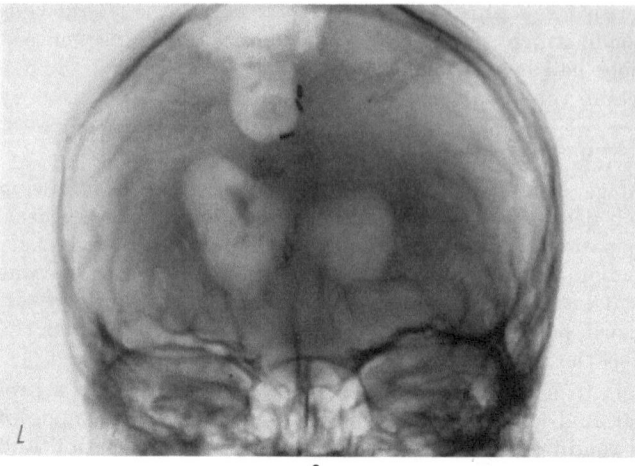

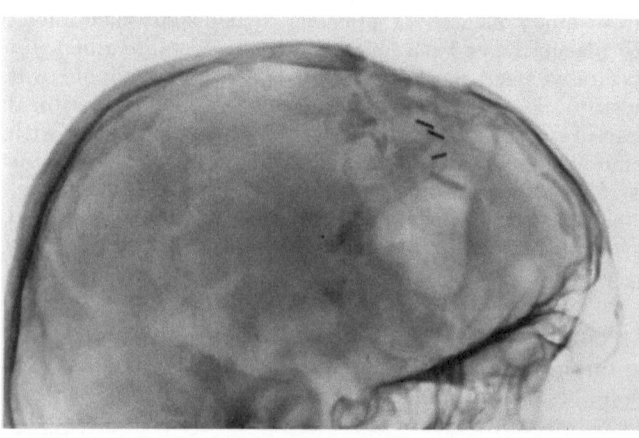

Fig. 46a and b. Air encephalogram (a.-p and a.-p. lateral views) in a case of penetrating missile wound in left frontal parasagittal region. Note smooth-edged trephine opening and 3 silver clips due to incomplete surgery in forward area. A number of deeply dislodged bone chips have been left behind. An air encephalography was performed 12 days after wounding, and shows the typical recess-like local dilatation of the adjoining anterior horn indicating local loss of brain tissue (1941)

be feared at surgical interventions at this stage, especially when radical excision of the abscess is attempted. A preliminary air encephalogram will provide valuable information as to the size and shape of the ventricles.

With intraventricular penicillin instillations now at hand, bacterial invasion of the lateral ventricles has lost part of its former grim outlook. GURDJIAN and WEBSTER (1948) have reported on successful treatment, by this method, of a pyocephalus of the lateral ventricle. There is a definite tendency on the part of the choroid plexus to seal off tightly any infected part of the lateral ventricle. This may result in a circumscribed intraventricular abscess amenable to successful surgical removal (CAIRNS et al., 1947). Apparently, the choroid plexus may react in a fashion comparable to that of the omentum under similar circumstances within the peritoneal cavity. To this phenomenon are closely related the localised forms

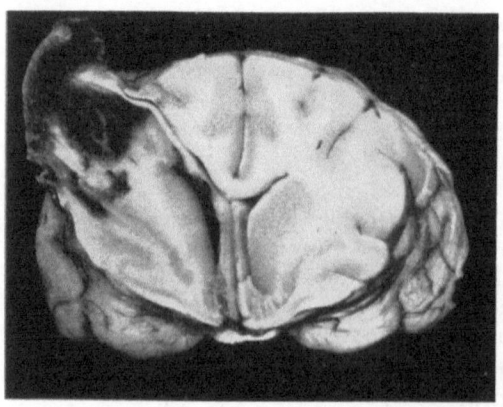

Fig. 47. This is from a series of experimental brain wounds in cats (IRSIGLER, 1942). In the animal the brain of which is shown above, a trephine opening, about 1 cm. in diameter, had been made under aseptic conditions, and the dura left open. The bone was not re-inserted, thus reproducing what TÖNNIS called ,,offene Knochenlücke". The scalp was closed by stitching it up. Within 9 days when the animal was sacrificed, a cerebral fungus of considerable size had developed and was enhanced by confluent haemorrhages and oedema. No infection was present. There is a deep-seated streaky bleed adjacent to the ventricle. Note slit-like elongation of the lateral ventricle projecting, eccentrically, into the fungating mass. The midline is deviated to the side of brain hernia. [From Zbl. Neurochir. 7, 27 (1942), Leipzig: J. A. Barth Verlag)

of partial hydrocephalus following penetrating wounds of the ventricles as described by CAIRNS and his coworkers in 1947.

11. Conclusion. Apropos surgical management of early brain abscess following penetrating missile injuries

The "octopus" type of drainage as introduced by TÖNNIS (1941) and his team during the influx of many cases of early brain abscess due to penetrating missile wounds, was designed to fulfill a twofold purpose: first, to keep open the missile track or abscess cavity so as to preclude purulent retention while the bottom of the abscess was allowed to granulate thus forming the "Wucherungszone" of SPATZ, and to approach gradually the level of the skin; secondly, and simultaneously, to restore, by reconstitution of the scalp and pericranium, the intracranial pressure dynamics as much as possible in order to provide for the infected brain wound near-normal conditions of blood supply and "tissue rest", the accepted prerequisits of all wound healing. To achieve this, tight closure around the tip of the drain by approximating the edges of the scalp had to be carried out.

The intrinsic efficacy of this method has been proved in many cases and often under most primitive circumstances (Fig. 41).

In a number of cases, however, this method of "tight" drainage proved to be inadequate because of too extensive loss of skin and dura mater (Fig. 42) preventing tight closure around the drainage tube, and because of the presence of multiloculated or collarstud abscesses; it also failed, of course, in cases of unsuspected abscess within the adjoining cerebral lobe (case 2.2.3, p. 73).

With no penicillin available in 1941, local chemotherapy was confined to frosting of the scalp wound and surface of fungus with sulphonamide powder, such as marfanil-prontalbin powder which was extensively used even in the forward echelons. Advent of penicillin (CAIRNS, 1944) resulted in a marked drop of the death rate in brain abscess (JOOMA et al., 1951) albeit, it should be remembered that, with the aid of sulphonamides alone, primary healing of infected brain wounds even on delayed treatment has been achieved as indicated by the impressive series of SCHWARZ and ROULHAC (1945).

The shortcomings of rubber drainage of the early brain abscess were well realized during the last war. To avoid these, PEIPER[1] has inaugurated the rubber sponge tamponade, and reported a death rate of 17% in an unselected series of 583 infected brain wounds. KRÜGER (1950) by combining PEIPER's tamponade with rigid rubber drainage and closure of the scalp, provided a "balanced" pressure system designed to put the brain to rest during the critical post-operative period; KRÜGER reported on 4 successful operations by this method, two of which were carried out on early brain abscesses due to penetrating injuries.

RIECHERT suggested, as early as 1942, covering of chronic irreducible brain fungi by mobilized skin-galea flaps which were shifted and sutured over the herniating mass, while two rubber tubes permitted of drainage through relaxation incisions. At such late stage rupture of the lateral ventricle forming a diverticulum beneath the bone opening was, in the pre-penicillin era, a real and everlasting danger to the patient's life. The inherent problem, so far, remains the same: surgical management of the heavily infected, suppurating and abscessing brain wound. "Open" treatment by tamponade, widely used in World War I, was again advocated by O'CONNELL in 1948 in the form of a modified water-proof MIKULICZ's tamponade.

Exteriorization of the abscess cavity, as inaugurated by KING in 1924, and revived by BROWDER in 1943 in the treatment of cranio-cerebral wounds was successfully combined with temporary dural grafting by WEBSTER and his coworkers (1946[a]) in the management of early brain abscesses due to war injuries during 1945. In the same series of 33 cases the

---

[1] PEIPER, H.: Dtsch. med. Wschr. 349 (1944); Chirurg 16, 138 (1944). Vide also footnote on p. 65.

authors have included 5 cases in which scalp closure (with or without mobilization) was performed after excision and complete enucleation of an underlying abscess; three cases were failures.

Evidently, the ideal treatment to be attempted in every case would be tight and permanent scalp closure after excision of the abscess including its capsule — as much of it as has formed at the time — followed by temporary[1] or final dural graft and adequate chemotherapy, systemic, intrathecal, and local, the latter through small rubber or plastic tubes (CAIRNS, 1944) or through the scalp (WEBSTER et al., 1946a).

Radical resection of infected brain wounds at a very early stage presenting with fulminating cerebritis and fungation, followed by open method of treatment has been proposed by MEIROWSKY and HARSH III during the Korea campaign (1953). Among 17 cases, so treated, there were only 3 deaths, ventricular involvement being present in no less than 65% of their cases. Repeated lumbar punctures or continuous spinal drainage were employed to maintain low intracranial pressure during the period of open after-care which extended, in some cases, to 82 days.

It is obvious that the intricate and time-consuming post-operative manoeuvres as described by the authors can be carried out only in a fully equipped unit abounding in time as well as surgical and nursing staff. It is remarkable that the American authors were provided with such facilities in a mobile neurosurgical team in the advanced area.

III. Late traumatic abscess of the brain
(See Table 7)

Experiences during the last war have amply confirmed that increasing thoroughness in primary debridement of penetrating brain wounds followed by complete wound closure results in lowering the rate of late traumatic abscesses of the brain. LEMKE, at the beginning of the war, reported on 11 late abscesses seen in a single unit by the end of 1941. Compared to this figure, the 14 cases reported by CAIRNS et al. in 1947 in a survey on delayed complications after head wounds, appears to be a low incidence. Obviously, chemotherapy began to play, during the war, an increasingly important rôle in the prevention of late complications. It is therefore significant that the majority of cases in CAIRN's series were treated before the advent of penicillin.

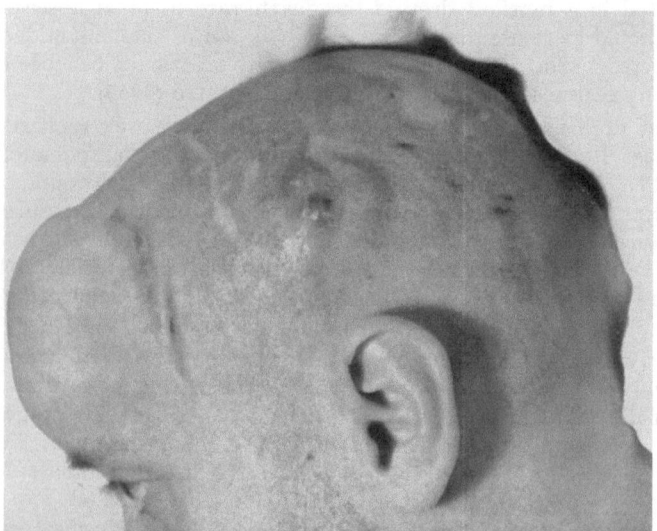

Fig. 48. Late abscess in left hemisphere following primary debridement and closure following deep laceration to the left frontal lobe, one year previously. Note bulge over trephined area and discharging sinus within scar behind. (Case 2.3.1)

1. Diagnosis

Among the important *diagnostic features* indicative of a late traumatic abscess of the brain are the following: presence of a discharging sinus or sinuses in the region of the scar left by the previous injury. This point is exemplified by the first two cases in the above series; a bulge or

---

[1] A temporary water-tight occluding dressing made of gauze and Zinc paste has been used by LEMKE in 1941.

increasing tension over the trephined area (Fig. 48); a flare-up of the clinical picture; presence of bone chips on the X-rays indicating incomplete previous debridement. If, as shown in case 2.3.4, both metallic and bone fragments are present a late abscess is more likely to be found related to the indriven bone. Small metal fragments appear to be less harmful. CAIRNS, in his series of 14 cases mentioned above, had only one chronic abscess around a retained missile. In our case 2.3.7, operated upon in 1944, a small missile fragment was found in the operative specimen within the abscess cavity; it had lodged there silently since the First World War. CAIRNS and DONALD, in 1934, removed a huge parietal abscess from a patient wounded in the First World War.

2. Air studies

Air studies, usually by ventricular tap, may considerably aid in localising the abscess. There was a marked shift of the ventricular system in the 4 patients in the above series

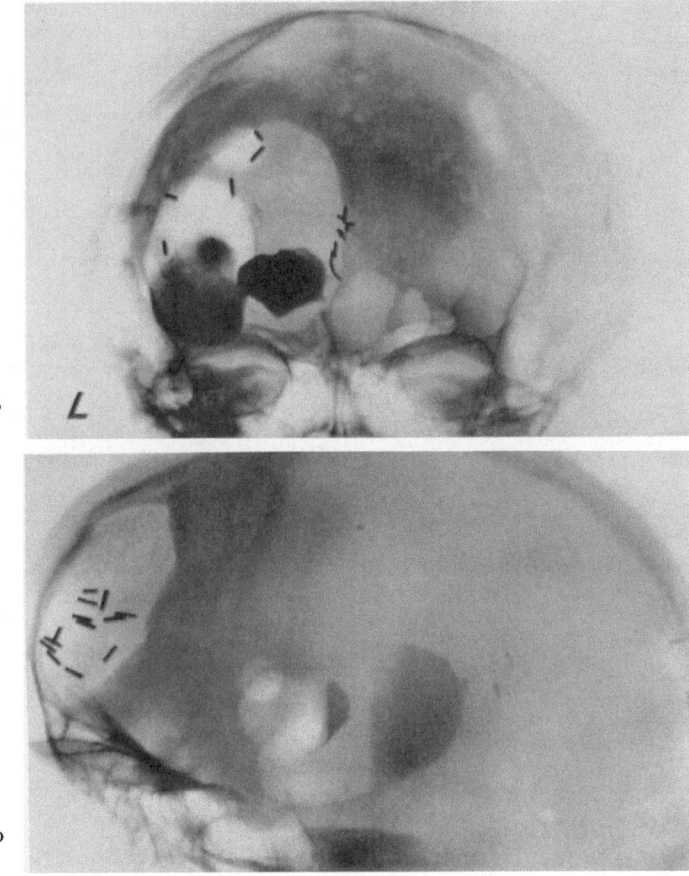

a

L

b

Fig. 49 a and b. Same patient as in previous figure. The multiloculated abscess has been visualized by air and thoro-trast (a.-p. and a.-p. lateral views). Note thick layer of pus within the greater cavity, between the thorotrast which outlines the bottom of the cavity, and air. The smooth-edged trephine opening and the silver clips are due to the debridement one year previously. The abscess was radically excised and the patient recoverd but was left with pronounced personality changes. (Case 2.3.1)

who had ventriculography, in addition to local distortion indicating pressure on that part of the lateral ventricle adjoining the abscess. In the 2 cases presenting with an abscess many years after their injuries, the ventricular displacement indicated that, quite in

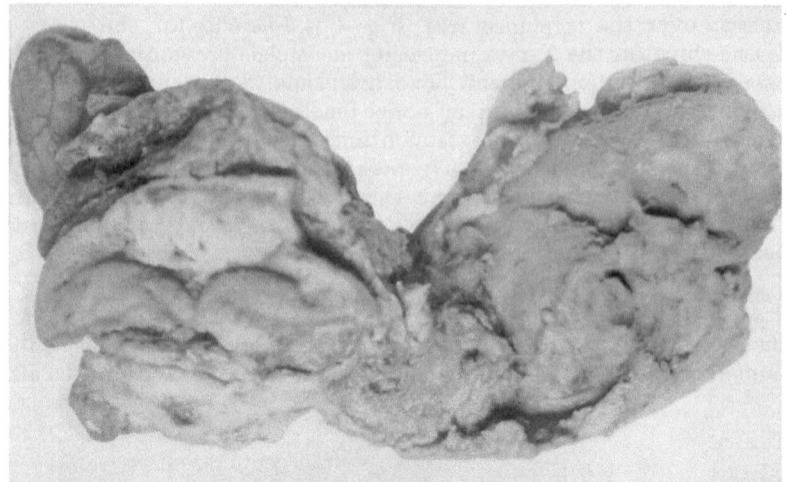

Fig. 50

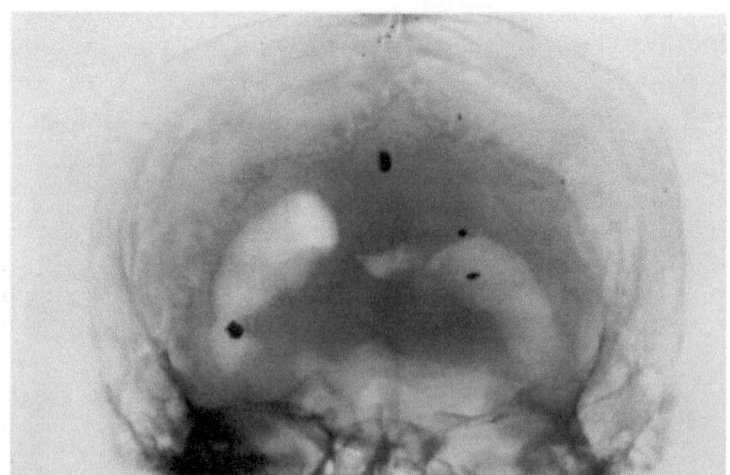

Fig. 51 a

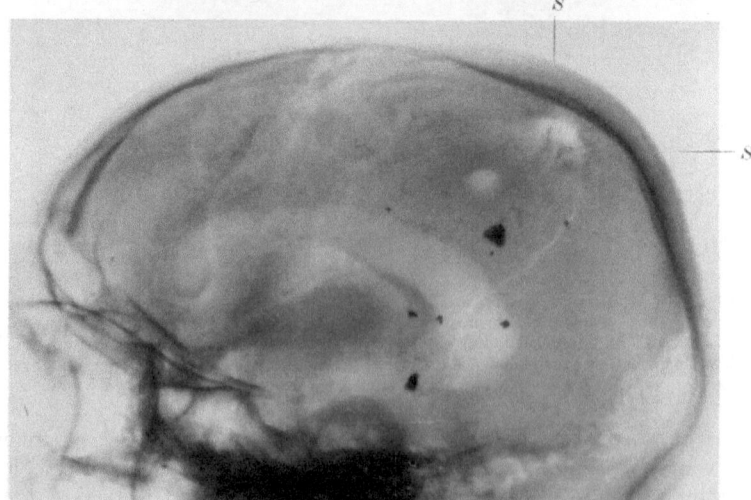

Fig. 51 b

Table 7. *Synopsis of 7 cases of late post-traumatic cerebral abscess*

Case no.	Interval from injury to clinical flare-up	Clinical findings	Operation	Outcome
2.3.1	Primary and complete debridement of penetrating injury to left frontal lobe, one year previously	Chronic lobotomy syndrome with episodes of behavioural derangement. Scalp bulging over trephined area (Fig.48), discharging sinus within scar. Multilocular abscess in left hemisphere visualized with thorotrast (Fig. 49)	Radical excision including capsule	Recovered from intracranial suppuration, was left with a depressed scar over bony defect; no change in mental state
2.3.2	Unknown	2 discharging sinuses within scar on left	Radical excision including capsule	Unknown
2.3.3	Unknown	Late abscess in left temporal lobe	Radical removal including meningo-cerebral scar (Fig. 50)	Unknown
2.3.4	Unknown	Late abscess in left postero-parietal area related to in-driven bone spicules	*Air encephalogram* showed marked shift to left and displacement of posterior part of left lateral ventricle (Fig.51)	Unknown
2.3.5	$6^1/_2$ $(10^1/_2?)$ weeks	Flare-up with left hemiparesis, right 6th nerve weakness, incipient papilloedema and pleocytosis in lumbar fluid. X-rays shew one retained bone fragment. Longitudinal scar over right parietal region, healed up p.pr. intention	*Ventriculography:* shift to left with tilt of septum pellucidum to right; saddle-like depression of roof of left lateral ventricle. Aspiration and drainage (nearly 3 fluid ounces of thick pus were withdrawn)	Unknown
2.3.6	Injury in childhood	Operative scar in left parietal region. Acute signs of raised intracranial pressure since 2 weeks ago. *Ventriculography:* shift to right and depression of roof of left lateral ventricle	Radical excision of para-sagittal abscess including dense capsule which ruptured during removal and contained viscous greenish pus with an offensive smell. Sulphonamide powder applied topically. Operative specimen see Fig. 52	Primary healing. Slow recovery from hemiparesis by the 4th week after operation. No late sequelae recorded
2.3.7	Nearly 30 years. (Missile wound during 1st world war)	Wound of entrance in right parietal region; retained shell fragment in left parietal lobe. Recently, acute signs of raised intracranial pressure developed. *Ventriculography:* marked shift to the right	Radical excision of deep-seated parasagittal abscess with an irregular capsule attached to the falx cerebri. Capsule ruptured during operation, contained creamy pus. Missile fragment found inside abscess cavity. Operative specimen see Fig. 53	Died 2 days following operation; microscopy revealed lymphoplasmacellular meningitis (Dr. EICKE, Berlin)

keeping with the clinical history, the formation of the cerebral abscess to such proportions as to result in an expanding mass, was a matter of recent development. It is noteworthy also that in either case the presence of a considerable amount of mesenchymal scar tissue around the abscess as evinced by the operative specimens did not prevent a ventricular shift.

In the above series the question of purulent cerebral thrombophlebitis which occasionally may lead to contralateral displacement of the lateral ventricles (PENNYBACKER,

---

Fig. 50. Operative specimen of a radically removed late abscess from the left temporal lobe. Attached to the abscess an extensive meningo-cerebral scar can be seen. War injury. (Case 2.3.3)

Fig. 51a and b. Air encephalogram (p.-a and lateral views) in a patient with a late abscess in left parietal lobe following missile injury. Note shift across midline and displacement of posterior part of left lateral ventricle. It can be seen that the abscess is related to a cluster of indriven bone spiculae (S) whereas small metallic foreign bodies lodge in either hemisphere, one of them alongside the falx cerebri. (Case 2.3.4)

1945), did not arise and it was not found in any of the cases. Finally, the air encephalogram will be found contributory in differentiating a late abscess from a traumatic cyst communicating with the ventricle. An example of this is illustrated in Fig. 54.

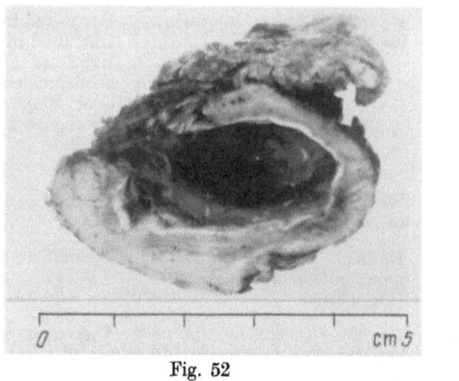
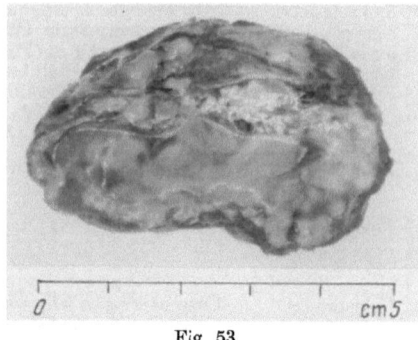

Fig. 52   Fig. 53

Fig. 52. Operative specimen (cut open) of a radically removed late traumatic abscess in left parietal lobe near the falx cerebri. Injury in childhood. Although the capsule ruptured during excision the wound healing was per primary intention. Note the dense capsule. The abscess had been clinically silent until 2 weeks prior to admission (Case 2. 3.6)

Fig. 53. Operative specimen (cut open to show synovia-like capsule) of a late traumatic abscess in left parietal lobe. Note bulk of scar tissue surrounding the abscess which contained creamy pus and a shell fragment that had lodged there since World War I. (Case 2.3.7)

3. Capsule formation

The formation of a well-defined capsule around the brain abscess probably takes less time than was previously thought. BUCY (1938), expressing a widely held view stated that encapsulation requires about 4 to 6 weeks. According to LE BEAU (1946), three weeks is long enough in many instances; this agrees with my own experiences. Surely, a capsule like the one in case 2.3.6 (Fig. 52) would hardly form within 2 to 3 weeks as the history might suggest, and one is led to the conclusion that in this case (and possibly in others, too) recrudescence of a dormant infection has taken place within an old cerebral cicatrix. This mode of development has been suggested, on good grounds, by CAIRNS et al. in 1947[a].

It has often been pointed out that the *pyogenic membrane surrounding* a brain abscess may be of varying thickness, thin or even absent at places, especially in the deeper layers near the lateral ventricle. LE BEAU feels justified to classify this type of chronic brain abscess as a type of its own which he calls "irregular" abscess. In shelling out such abscesses, rupture of the capsule with or without disruption of the ventricular ependyma is likely to occur; contamination of the field including the subdural space usually follows.

On exposing the parasagittal abscess in case 2.3.7 the first impression was not unlike that of a parasagittal meningioma. Even the vascular pattern of the cortex surrounding the lesion was thought consistent with that of a subcortical tumour. Consequently, the excision of this abscess followed the lines in general use for removing a parasagittal meningioma. Apparently, fibrous tissue overlying a late abscess, may produce circumscribed depression of the brain surface. It also predisposes to recurrent infection — certainly an additional hint at the advisability of careful surgical excision of all cicatricial residues within the brain substance at the very first surgical attack on any penetrating brain injury (Fig. 50).

4. Treatment

As to the treatment, the present series is too limited and follow-up knowledge too scanty for final assessment. In our series of 7 cases radical excision of the abscess was carried out five times; of these, one patient died, two survived and in two the final outcome is unknown. There is little doubt that radical excision so as to include all fibrous strands and appendages of collagenous scar tissue is the method of choice both from the point of view of preventing recrudescent suppuration as well as post-traumatic epilepsy. Here, war

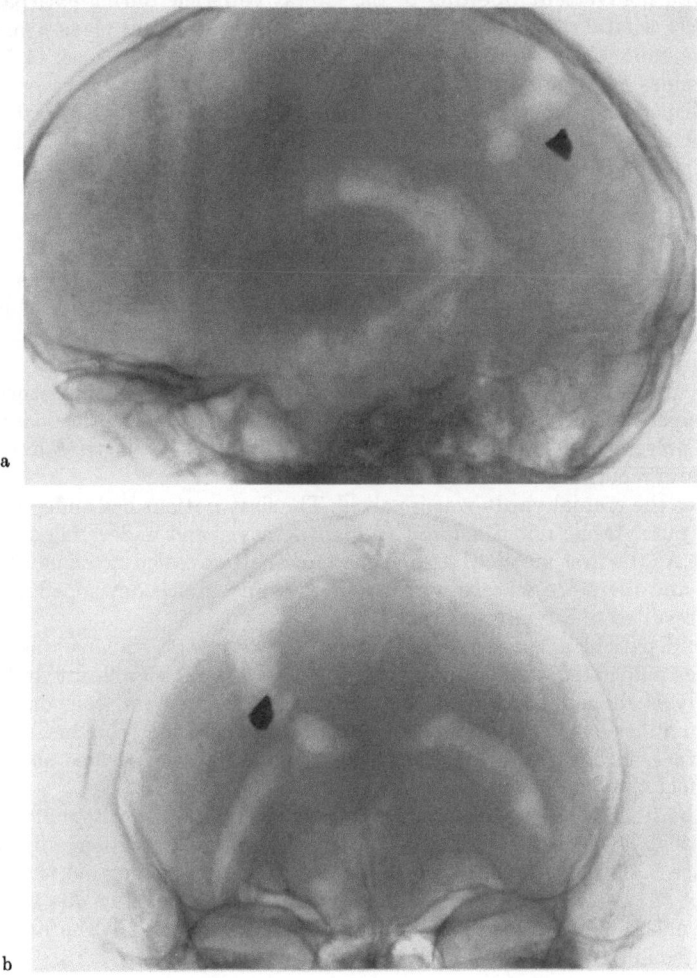

Fig. 54 a and b. Air encephalogram (p.-a and p.-a lateral views) in a youngster who was shot while engaged in play. The missile entered the cranium above the root of his nose to lodge in the right parietal lobe. No infection developed. The air studies revealed an intracerebral cyst related to the retained metallic body, and communicating with the subarachnoid space. Note absence of space-occupying lesion and ventricular dilatation although the missile, quite possibly, traversed the ventricular system. If the bullet, after hitting the tabula interna, re-entered the brain this would mean a ricochet type of trajectory. The bullet was removed successfully including surrounding scar tissue

surgery has wisely and successfully followed the steps of peace-time experience. KRÖNLEIN, in 1910, was the first to succeed in radical removal of three brain abscesses. The modern method, now in general use, is due to VINCENT (1936) and his followers (LE BEAU, 1946).

BLÜMEL and KRAUS[1] recently reported a primary mortality of 19% in 26 posttraumatic abscesses treated by operation and with antibiotics.

During the last war LEMKE, to my knowledge, was the first to apply VINCENT's method successfully to late abscesses due to missile wounds of the brain. By the end of 1941,

[1] Zbl. Neurochir. **19**, 273 (1959).

LEMKE reported on eleven late abscesses radically excised, with only one death. A later report by the same author (1944) deals with 20 patients, three of whom died.

LEMKE's and the experiences of many others later have shown that rupture of the capsule and even inadvertent opening of the lateral ventricle during extirpation do not necessarily imply a fatal outcome. Obviously, chemotherapy here plays a major part in surgical management. LEMKE's results are the more remarkable because, in 1941, he had only sulphonamides at his disposal. In the later development of such cases repeated air studies are indispensable whenever, following brain injury of the penetrating type, the necessity arises to assess size and shape of the ventricular system, and/or to rule out a suspected expanding lesion.

IV. Brain abscess by continuity

In this section we will be concerned with two cases only. The one was seen by the writer in 1943, the other in 1949 — a short but significant interval during which penicillin came into general use. Consequently, one may expect the two cases to reflect the advances in chemotherapy achieved within the short period of six years.

Centripetal spread of infection in either case is apparent from their histories and confirmed by the operative findings. It is worth mentioning that in neither case a subdural empyema was present; this was especially expected in the second patient but ruled out, first by exploratory burr holes and later at craniotomy.

In both cases the cranial vault was involved. The first patient had suffered a depressed fracture of the outer table, not disclosed on plain X-rays, and underlying a purulent discharging sinus. At the first surgical attack the bone had revealed no signs of infection to the naked eye and therefore was re-wired; however, an osteitis developed soon after the operation and resulted in a recurrent scalp sinus.

In the second patient a local osteomyelitis of the temporal squama was apparent on exposure; it was associated with a subaponeurotic abscess. A significant finding and one which obviously is related to the continuous spread of infection from outside was the presence of firm adhesions between the dura mater and the underlying brain cortex at the site of the abscess; in both patients, these adhesions had to be severed sharply in order to free and reflect the dura mater.

Finally, in both cases the abscess was within the subcortical white matter and roofed by a thin cortical layer which, in case 2.4.1 was removed together with the abscess (Fig. 55); in case 2.4.2 the cortical layer was sacrificed after shelling out the abscess. The osteomyelitis of the temporal bone in the second case was possibly due to a preceding frontal sinus or mastoid infection; however (although not suggested by the history), a bloodborne infection could not be entirely ruled out in this patient.

Case 2.4.1. Brain abscess underneath draining scalp sinus due to blunt trauma to the head. Radical excision of well-delineated mass which, at first sight, was thought to be a subcortical glioma. Transient improvement was followed by purulent cerebritis probably due to recurrent infection of the bone flap.

This was a man of 37 who, $2^{1}/_{2}$ months prior to admission, had suffered an injury to the right side of his head when he was hit by a falling brick. He had not been knocked unconcious and even tried to continue with his work. He was sent to a hospital where he stayed for 5 weeks. While he was in the hospital, he noted episodes of paraesthesiae and a gradually progressing weakness of his left arm. Following electrical treatment he developed jacksonian twitchings involving his left hand and the left half of his face. The twitchings recurred once or twice and eventually led to his transfer to the Berlin Clinic. He presented with complaints of painful tingling in his left hand and with an indrawn scar firmly adherent to the underlying bone, in the right postero-parietal region. At this site, there was a sero-purulent discharging sinus of the scalp. Because of the discharge and in the abscence of pressure signs, surgery was postponed for 3 weeks. An air encephalogram revealed, on the p.a. view, a displacement of the lateral ventricles to the left with a considerable depression of the roof of the right ventricle beneath the falx cerebri. A right carotid angiography delineated an expanding mass in the right postero-parietal area which, because of its paucity in vascular channels, was interpreted in terms of a cystic tumour, perhaps a subcortical astrocytoma. The history of jacksonian seizures, both sensory and motor, was thought to support this tentative diagnosis. No signs of a subdural effusion related to the discharging sinus were present on the angiogram.

With the patient in the face-down position, an osteoplastic flap crossing the midline, was turned down in the right parietal region under local anaesthesia. It was found that the tabula externa was slightly depressed whereas the internal table was intact. The dura mater was slack and was found to be adherent to the brain. It was opened and reflected across the longitudinal sinus to the left. The rolandic veins were identified and the greater part of a convolution which was held to be the posterior central gyrus was found conspicuously broadened and somewhat bulging. Its colour was slightly pale and this seemed to indicate an abnormal blood supply and/or infiltration by abnormal tissue. When gently palpated, the convolution was felt to be soft as compared to the surrounding normal brain. Piecing together the clinical features and the operative findings a diagnosis

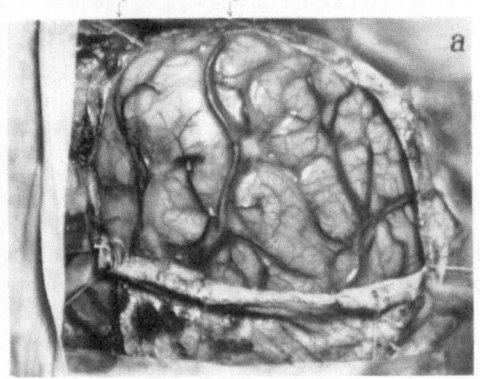

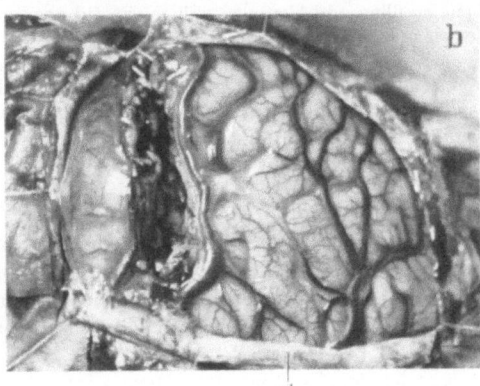

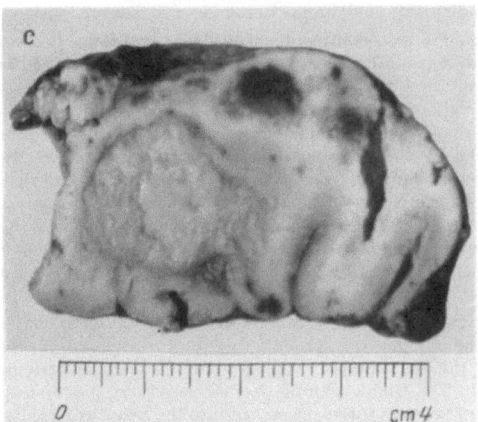

Fig. 55a and b are photos taken during craniotomy over right rolandic area. Dura (d) opened and reflected across sagittal sinus which marks the lower margin of the operative field in both pictures.

Compare the convolutional pattern before (a) and after excision (b) of the abnormal gyrus between two rolandic veins (r_1 and r_2). On exposure we thought we were dealing with a subcortical glioma.

The excisum is shown in c. A circumscribed roundish mass, not quite one inch in diameter, and with a caseous centre, is seen on the cut surface and appears to be removed together with surrounding healthy-looking brain tissue. The lesion turned out to be an abscess.

In spite of continuous spread of infection from the scalp as suggested by the history in this case, neither a subdural effusion nor local meningitis were present.

(Case 2.4.1)

N.B. Scale at bottom of C is in mms.

of a small subcortical glioma was made and the convolution excised in toto by cautery down to a depth of approximately 4 cm. from the surface (Fig. 55). The cut surface of the operative specimen confirmed that the lesion was well circumscribed and apparently had been removed completely. There was no bleeding and the entire operation including re-wiring of the bone and re-suturing of the scalp took not more than 90 minutes.

Under the microscope, the lesion turned out to be an abscess with an onion-like stratified pyogenic membrane surrounding a caseous centre.

The patient stood the operation well but was left with a flaccid paralysis of the left side of his body which, however, rapidly improved from the 2nd day on, the distal parts of the limbs being the last ones to recover. On the 6th day the muscle tone and the tendon reflexes on the left were found increased as compared to the right and an ankle clonus became elicitable while BABINSKI's sign on the left remained equivocal. During the 3rd post-operative week the patient's condition started deteriorating again; his hemiparesis worsened and a striking change in his personality became apparent. Whereas the operative incision itself healed up per primary union the centre of the scalp flap around the scar broke down to lay open an osteitic bone flap. Ventriculography confirmed another expanding mass on the right.

Under local anaesthesia, the flap was raised again and the bone lifted up; its under-surface was covered with suppurating granulations. The dura mater was tight and torn, and underneath, a purulent exudate within the pia-arachnoid was present. Adjacent to the site of previous excision the brain was pulpy, changed into a mass of debris and pus. A badly defined brain abscess was opened up and two glove drains were inserted and issued through the defect in the scalp. The field was then frosted with sulphonamide powder and the scalp flap re-sutured. The patient succumbed soon afterwards with signs of spreading purulent cerebritis. Pus from the abscess yielded no growth on culture.

Comment. Misinterpretation of a brain abscess for a neoplasm is not infrequent. It happened to KRÖN-LEIN (1910) in one of his successfully removed brain abscesses. In BUCY's (1938) words: "Like many other neurosurgeons, we have had the experience of enucleating an encapsulated abscess under the mistaken impression that we were dealing with a tumour", and subsequently gave an instance in point. The difficulties in differential diagnosis have been discussed at some length by PENNYBACKER in 1945 who suggested exploratory brain needling and biopsy, as well as carotid angiography. That the latter may be misleading is exemplified by our case.

In view of the history and the presence of a discharging scalp sinus an extradural or subdural abscess appeared likely; both were ruled out by angiography. It is hard to see how the angiogram could be of assistance in differential diagnosis between a cystic neoplasm and a brain abscess.

The recurrence of intradural suppuration which eventually gave rise to purulent cerebritis in spite of radical excision of the well walled-off abscess of Fig. 55 is probably due either to the presence of yet another abscess overlooked at the first surgical intervention, or, and more likely, to intradural infection spreading from osteitis of the bone flap.

The following case history will be mentioned here only briefly since both KRAYENBÜHL and WEBER in 1952, and WEBER in his monograph in 1957 have discussed the case more fully. It is included here because the present writer had the privilege to see this patient at the Neurosurgical Clinic in Zürich in 1949 and to assist at the operation which was performed by Dr. G. WEBER.

Case 2.4.2. Abscess of the right temporal lobe, possibly following frontal sinusitis 6 weeks previously, and ushered in by local osteomyelitis of the temporal plate. Aspiration and chemotherapy unsatisfactory. Craniectomy and radical excision including friable capsule and surrounding softened brain. Recovery.

This was a young watch-maker of 24 years who had taken ill with complaints of headache and fever 6 weeks prior to admission; the attack was thought to be due to a frontal sinusitis. At first, he responded well to treatment with sulphonamides but soon the headache returned and he started vomiting. He was taken to a hospital because of a tender fluctuant swelling in the right temporal fossa, and signs of meningitis. Additionally, a left-sided hemiparesis became apparent and a homonymous hemianopia to the left was noted. During the following three weeks the patient was given penicillin by the intramuscular and intrathecal routes. He became increasingly lethargic and eventually was referred to the clinic. An abscess was entered in the right hemisphere with the brain needle and visualized with air on the X-rays. The abscess was the size of an orange occupying the greater part of the right temporal lobe. 20 ml. of pus were withdrawn in which staphylococcus aureus was found to be present. 10,000 units of penicillin were instilled into the abscess cavity, and 15,000 units intrathecally; sulphonamides were given systemically. In spite of this, he lapsed into a deep coma and the left side of his body became paralysed completely.

A temporal craniectomy was now carried out on the right side and a circumscribed osteomyelitis of the temporal squama was found. At this site a drop of extradural pus was present. The dura mater was firmly adherent to the brain surface; after freeing and reflecting the dura the thin wall of a brain abscess underlying the eroded bone was opened and pus removed by suction. The friable capsule was dissected out piece-meal; the surrounding softened brain was sucked away gently and two polythene drains put into the resultant cavity. The wound was closed in layers, including the dura mater; the diseased bone flap was not re-inserted. Chemotherapy was continued for 21 days. The patient recovered, save for an hemianopic field defect to the left, diminished visual acuity in the right eye, and occasional epileptiform seizures.

Comment. The fortunate outcome in this case undoubtedly was chiefly due to adequate chemotherapy before, during, and after the two surgical interventions of which the first — aspiration — proved ineffective in preventing progress in neurological signs. The result of radical surgery was the more remarkable since the excision was carried out during the period of rapidly increasing intracranial pressure on the one hand and incomplete encapsulation of the abscess on the other, necessitating, after piece-meal removal of a defective pyogenic membrane, additional removal by suction of adjoining brain tissue which showed signs of bacterial invasion. Contamination of the resultant cavity was kept under control by penicillin instillations through thin polythene drains. The bacterial agent involved was a staphylococcus. In marked contrast to the first case this was an acute brain abscess as evinced by a tight dura mater and clinical signs of rapid progression. The case, I think, demonstrates conclusively the effectiveness of radical surgery supplemented by modern chemotherapy, during the stage of formation and incomplete demarcation of a brain abscess.

C. The otogenous class

The following discussion refers to the synoptic Table 8 in which details of individual cases are summarized.

1. The supratentorial group (cases 3.1—3.5)

There are five cases in this group which comprises otogenous abscesses seated in one of the temporal lobes. The left hemisphere was involved twice, the right hemisphere three times. There were three children in the group. One of the adults was seen in consultation at, and remained throughout on, the ENT. ward, whereas the other adult patient was transferred from that ward to the neurosurgical ward with the established diagnosis of left temporal lobe abscess. In both cases the visual fields were not reported by the aural surgeon, and lack of co-operation precluded charting of the fields in the three children. It is owing to these circumstances that the important neurological sign of visual field defect does not appear among the clinical features in the present series.

The incidence of supratentorial abscesses of otitic origin has long been reported as being considerably higher than the incidence of infratentorial suppurations of the same etiology. ADSON (1938) in cases of presumed otogenous abscess with conflicting or equivocal symptoms and signs suggested exploration of the temporal lobe before turning to the cerebellum. CAWTHORNE (1945) reported a ratio of incidence of 3:1 in favour of the supratentorial group. In the above series there were five temporal lobe abscesses as against one situated in the cerebellum.

Returning to the clinical syndrome, it should be mentioned that in case 3.5 where the the abscess was located in the speech representing hemisphere, the mixed type of aphasia was recorded with paraphasiae, difficulty in repeating sentences and words, and in giving the names of familiar objects when shown to the patient. He was able to indicate correctly right and left but soon became confused when asked to identify one of his fingers. Since there was no acalculia the diagnosis of a true GERSTMANN's syndrome was not warranted.

It has been pointed out that in the majority of cases the original ear infection has become chronic by the time the first signs of intracranial suppuration appear. This is borne out by five of the six otogenous abscesses listed above in all of which the otitis or its equivalent, the otogenous meningitis preceded the onset of the abscess in the brain by a period ranging from 4 weeks to 9 months.

It is significant also that the brain abscess as a rule made its appearance without distinct signs of an acute flare-up of the local ear infection. Only in case 3.5 a left temporal abscess became apparent to the aural surgeon during the acute stage following radical mastoidectomy performed a fortnight previously. This abscess was aspirated and drained on the 13th day after the mastoid operation while the wound was still discharging copiously. It also seems significant that in this case signs of a recurrent brain abscess appeared while the discharge through the track connecting the abscess cavity with the mastoid wound, became conspicuously less.

Hemiparesis of the limbs and/or the face may be a significant and comparatively early feature in temporal lobe abscess of otitic origin. It was noted in case 3.3 apparently as the first sign heralding intracranial complication three weeks after the ear infection which, by this time, had settled down under conservative treatment.

In patient 3.4 who was under sulphonamide treatment, a fleeting middle ear infection was followed by a lucid interval of short duration; then suddenly acute signs of increased pressure and tentorial displacement developed and were associated with a contralateral hemiparesis. Also, in case 3.5 a right facial weakness was noticed when the patient was first seen neurologically four weeks after drainage of a left temporal lobe abscess.

Apart from the patient just mentioned where a "dry" spinal tap was followed by a series of jacksonian fits involving the ipsilateral half of the body, only in case 3.10 left-sided jacksonian convulsions of the adversive type were noted; in fact, they led to the patient's

Table 8. *Synopsis of 13 case histories in the otogenous class*

Case no.	Clinical	Site of abscess or lesion	Operation	Outcome
3.1	Mastoidectomy 8 weeks prior to admission	Left temporal	Enucleation after tap, with part of covering dura, see Fig. 58	Wound healing p. pr. Recovered
3.2 (child)	Otitic meningitis 9 months prior to admission	Right temporal	Right temporal lobectomy, dura and brain very tight, two deep-seated abscesses one of which ruptured during excision (Fig. 57)	Died from purulent meningitis over right convexity and multiple abscesses scattered throughout right hemisphere
3.3 (child)	Expectant treatment of otitis 7 weeks prior to admission; 3 weeks following otitis left-sided weakness noted	Right occipital	Occipital lobectomy incl. encapsulated dumb-bell abscess (Fig. 59)	Wound healing p. pr. Recovered
3.4 (infant)	Otitis media and pleocytosis, treated with sulphonamides, 4 weeks prior to admission; then lucid interval followed by drowsiness and neck rigor, right pupil dilated, weakness on left, bilateral extensor response	Right temporal	Huge subcortical abscess aspirated through burr hole; creamy pus with offensive smell; g + cocci and bacilli. Soft rubber drainage	Died from suppurative encephalitis spreading into frontal lobe
3.5	Left radical mastoidectomy was followed by purulent discharge from the wound; 13 days later aspiration and drainage of left temporal lobe abscess; marked pleocytosis in the lumbar fluid	Left temporal	Pat. lingered on ENT. ward, with profuse foul discharge from the mastoid wound. Finally, a papilloedema on the left developed and air studies revealed shift to right	10 weeks after drainage of abscess a recurrent abscess developed in left temporal lobe, and another operative attempt was made by the aural surgeon which was followed by a fatal meningitis
3.6	Admitted with chronic otitis media on right; ? brain abscess	Pyocephalus internus (bilat.)	On mastoidectomy an extradural abscess was found; dura tight, not incised. After temporary improvement pyrexia and stupor, right pupil dilated and fixed, eye deviation to left, right 6th n. paresis, stertorous breathing, lumbar fluid turbid. Tracheotomy. Ventricular tap: flocculent pus with foul smell on either side	Died despite ventricular drainage and penicillin, 5 days after admission; no autopsy conceded
3.7	Admission in deep coma, with purulent discharge from right ear, central perforation in right drum. Fundi normal, left knee jerk increased, bilateral ankle clonus. Lumbar fluid clear and colourless, pressure 100 mms., 2 polymorphs. Air studies: doubtful shift to left. Tentative diagnosis of right temporal lobe abscess was made. (History of purulent mastoiditis on right, 6 months previously)	So-called Otitic Hydrocephalus (?)	Trephine opening over right temple, needling for abscess negative; fluid in temporal horn clear and pulsatile; dura incised, temporal lobe appeared normal	Died 5 hrs. after subtemporal decompression, in deepening coma. *Necropsy:* Convolutions slightly flattened, no abscess, no meningitis, no ventricular shift or dilatation, no thrombosis or thrombophlebitis (to the naked eye)
3.8	Purulent discharge from left ear of one month's duration. Radical mastoidectomy performed, ivory bone, no abscess found.	Left subtentorial abscess suspected clinically	Exploratory burr holes over left cerebellum and left postero-temporal region; (Fig. 60); slack dura, needling for abscess negative;	Died following day. Necropsy: basal meningitis with thick exudate suggesting TB though no tb. bacilli were found on ZIEHL-NEELSEN

Table 8. (Continued)

Case no.	Clinical	Site of abscess or lesion	Operation	Outcome
	Meningitis developed[1], 6th n. weakness on right, hypotonia in left arm and leg, nystagmoid jerks in left eye, no field defect, no papilloedema. Left cerebellar abscess suspected		increased amounts of turbid fluid within ventricle and in subarachnoid pools	slides. Localised accumulation of fluid in left cerebello-pontine angle. Moderate internal hydrocephalus
3.9	Chronic discharge from right ear for several months. Recently became drowsy and complained of headache. Right cerebellar signs, bilateral papilloedema and neck rigidity, mild 6th n. paresis on right	Right cerebellar	Tap evacuation of cerebellar abscess, instillation of mixture of antibiotics, drainage for 7 days. Duration of procedure: about 45 min. Pus: g + cocci and g + and g − bacilli, no growth on culture	Went into status epil. and respiratory arrest for nearly 8 hrs, deep coma. Then recovered. Ventricular drainage, papilloedema slowly subsided. 8 weeks after operation: right deafness, weakness of right face and limbs; incoördinate gait, atrophy of right optic disc. Occipital and sacral pressure sores healing up per sec.
3.10	Injury to right temple 4 weeks prior to admission for left jacksonian fits merging into status. — Scar in front of right pinna, discharging sinus behind ear. Comminuted fracture of pars mastoidea. Left-sided weakness; angiography: no shift	Right mastoid	Exposure (Fig. 56) and debridement, hairs between fragments, dura covered with granulations but intact, mastoid cells suppurating, were curetted and loosely packed with strips of gauze	Pat. transferred to ENT. ward for radical mastoidectomy, died there from meningitis
3.11	Missile injury with retained shell fragment, entry left ear. Pat. aphasic and confused, no hemiparesis	Left ear	Early brain abscess drained 12th (?) day after wounding, cluster of bone chips left behind. Re-debridement and octopus drain inserted	Slow recovery, healing per sec.; track opened up by lumbar taps. 6 weeks after wounding granulating field
3.12	Admitted with concussion, X-rays negative. Chemotherapy from the onset. On 3rd day sudden pyrexia, neck rigor and severe pain in left ear without discharge. Lumbar fluid turbid and under raised pressure	Left mastoid bone	Left mastoidectomy 11 days following admission, fracture in the roof of the recessus epitympanicus with leak of CSF. flooding the mastoid cells[2]	Wound healing p. pr. Patient recovered fully and permanently
3.13	Assaulted and hit on left side of face, profuse watery discharge from left ear from the beginning and persisting for the ensuing 10 days. No neurological deficit. X-rays: vertical fissure in left temporal squama extending (?) into floor of middle fossa; scattered intracranial air bubbles, 4th ventricle outlined by air. Lumbar fluid blood-stained	Post-traumatic otorrhoea on left side, persisting	Repair 10 days after injury by osteoplastic temporal flap. Temporalis muscle bruised. Extradural approach alongside floor of middle fossa where a fracture line, close to the foramen spinae, was disclosed; dura protuded into fracture, clear fluid escaping through hole in dura. Brisk bleed from middle meningeal artery and superior petrosal sinus, controlled by cautery. Free graft from the temporalis fascia tucked in between dura and bone, and sealed off with oxycel. Flap re-sutured	Profuse CSF. leak continued postoperatively; complete facial paralysis and lagophthalmos on left. Herpetic eruption on left upper lip from 6th postoperative day on. Sensation loss in 3rd division of left trigeminal n. Spinal drainage failed, then pat. improved and dural leak subsided spontaneously and permanently. Left with left facial weakness and perforation of left ear drum

[1] *Lumbar fluid:* protein 136 mgm.-%; polymorphs 7,100; globulin +; sugar 39 mgm.-%; chlorides 550 mgm.-%. Culture yielded non-haemolytic streptococci, E. coli, and proteus.
[2] Operation performed by Dr. J. H. Hofmeyr.

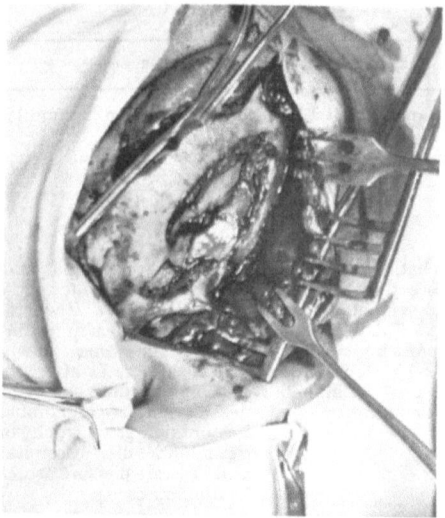

Fig. 56. Operative exposure of a comminuted fracture of the right mastoid region in a middle-aged woman who had been kicked by a horse 4 weeks previously, and was admitted with left-sided jacksonian fits. The mastoid cells were full of pus. Despite radical mastoidectomy the patient died from meningitis. Extradural and intra-cerebral abscesses were ruled out by carotid angiography. (Case 3.10)

transfer to the neurosurgical ward. Here, in addition to the convulsions, a left hemiparesis was found. On debridement of a comminuted right mastoid bone (Fig. 56) an extradural suppuration was present. A brain abscess, at this stage, was ruled out by carotid angiography. It is obvious from the postoperative course that in this case the surgical approach was inadequate and perhaps too late leaving behind infected mastoid cells as a focus of potential intracranial spread.

Evidently, such cases as 3.5 and 3.10 call for mutual understanding and close cooperation between the neurosurgeon and the aural surgeon. Unfortunately, one of the two finds himself from time to time confronted with an unforeseen situation which requires quick decision, and yet should be approached from a combined angle of view. So, in practice, an extradural abscess adjacent to mastoid infection in most cases will be handled by the otologist with whom then rests the responsibility of an additional intradural exploration. One would expect that such procedure should nowadays be deemed indispensable less frequently, not mentioning here the ill-advised and mis-directed needling from the mastoid wound for a suspected brain abscess either above or below the transverse sinus, a procedure which was mentioned, only a few years ago, among the causes of iatrogenic temporal lobe abscess.

The neurosurgeon when coming into play at a later stage will appreciate any hint on the part of the aural surgeon, as to the patency or obstruction of the lateral sinus and the appearance of the exposed part of the dura mater.

The results of surgical treatment in the above series may be summarized as follows: two of the three patients who had radical operation either by excision or lobectomy, survived;

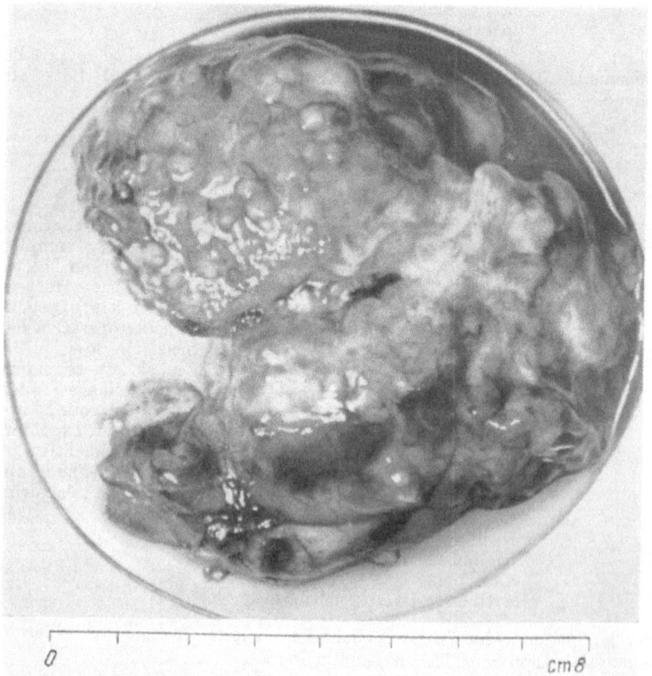

Fig. 57. Operative specimen containing two otogenous abscesses which were radically removed from the right temporal lobe in a child who, nine months before, had otitis media followed by an attack of meningitis. The child died from a recurrent meningitis over the right convexity. On the post mortem table, multiple abscesses were found to be present within the right cerebral hemisphere. (Case 3.2)

in the third case a right temporal lobectomy was carried out including two abscesses (Fig. 57) one of which ruptured during excision; additionally, the temporal horn was

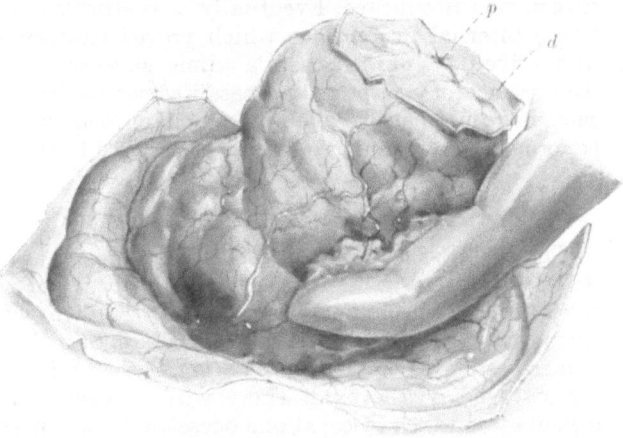

opened in this child giving rise to a meningitis over the corresponding convexity which obviously contributed to the fatal outcome due to the presence of multiple abscesses throughout the right hemisphere.

In the remaining two cases the abscess was aspirated and drained: the one through a formal approach by a separate opening in the temporal squama, the other from the mastoid wound. Both were failures. Case 3.4, a 2-year-old infant was treated with sulphathiazol and died from suppurative cerebritis extending into the adjacent frontal lobe. Case 3.5 appears to demonstrate conclusively that an otogenous temporal lobe abscess once it has passed the acute stage, should be treated as a lesion on its own account i.e. by direct attack according to accepted

Fig. 58. To show enucleation with finger of a multi-locular otogenous abscess from the left temporal lobe in a patient who had a mastoidectomy performed 8 weeks previously. Part of the dura mater (d) was firmly adherent to the surfacing capsule; it was circumcised and removed together with the abscess. At p the abscess had been tapped through the dura to relieve pressure before enucleation, and the hole in the dura was closed with a purse-string stitch. Wound healing was p. pr. (Case 3.1)

neurosurgical principles and through a clean field. This seems preferable even in the cases where a diseased and possibly isolated track between the mastoid wound and the abscess invites drainage along this track. It should be borne in mind that the attack from the mastoid

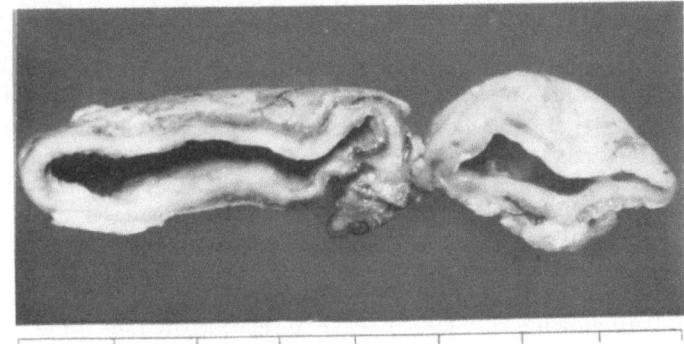

wound never allows radical excision and may fail (as it did in case 3.5) to maintain adequate drainage.

Except for case 3.2 where after temporal lobectomy multiple abscesses were found on the post mortem table within the remaining hemisphere no multiple or "distant" abscesses such as described by COURVILLE and NIELSEN[1] have been encountered in the present series. The cases 3.1 and 3.3 (Figs. 58 and 59 respectively) are two instances of dumb-bell temporal abscess of otitic origin which were successfully removed.

Fig. 59. Operative specimen of 2 encapsulated abscesses removed from the right occipital lobe in a child of 5 years who some 7 weeks previously had an attack of otitis media which was treated conservatively. One month after the onset of her illness a left-sided weakness became apparent and led to hospital admission. According to the history obtained the abscess was not older than 4 weeks. Note thickness of capsule. Wound healing after craniotomy and excision was p. pr. Scale at the bottom in cm. (Case 3.3)

2. Otogenous pyocephalus

Case 3.6, a native male, was the only instance of otogenous pyocephalus in the series. This complication developed in the presence of a longstanding aural infection which had

[1] West. J. Surg. **43**, 681 (1935).

been neglected until unmistakable signs of a more serious lesion appeared. Mastoidectomy at this late stage revealed an extradural collection of pus; the dura mater albeit under tension was not incised. Eventually, a ventricular tap established the diagnosis of a bilateral internal pyocephalus which proved fatal, in spite of intraventricular penicillin, within five days of the patient's admission to the hospital. As autopsy was not conceded the presence of a suspected abscess was not confirmed. There is but little doubt that the outcome would have been less disappointing had an early and radical mastoidectomy been performed or neurosurgical advice been called in at an earlier stage.

3. So-called otitic hydrocephalus

The middle-aged native man listed in Table 8 as case 3.7 deserves special discussion. He was admitted in deep coma with a history and evidence of right-sided mastoiditis of at least 6 months' duration. His right ear was still discharging and otoscopy revealed a large central perforation in the right drum. Except for the comatose state there were no signs of increased pressure and no choking of the optic discs. No convulsions were reported nor observed on the ward. There were no signs of meningitis either. The lumbar fluid pressure was taken twice; at one occasion it was reported to be 100 mm of water, whereas at a repeated tap, the pressure was found to be "high". The fluid was clear and contained 2 polymorphs per cmm. Exploratory craniotomy through the right temporal squama revealed no signs of undue tension on the dura and on the brain; presumably, foregoing lumbar taps had resulted in undue lowering of the intracranial pressure. Needling for an abscess was negative. The patient died without a definite diagnosis as to the nature of his intracranial pathology being established; nor did a careful dissection of the cranial cavity — partial necropsy only had been conceded — provide, to the naked eye, a satisfactory explanation. Apart from a moderate protrusion of the brain through the trephine opening there was no flattening of the convolutions nor coning present. The ventricles were within normal range as regards their size. There was no abscess or meningitis, and no thrombosis of the dural sinuses, and of the cortical and galenic systems.

Diagnosis of a so-called otitic hydrocephalus as originally conceived by SYMONDS in 1931, suggests itself in the case discussed here. In favour of this are the presence of a chronic discharging ear infection, absence of focal signs and a virtually normal lumbar fluid. Unfortunately, we are not quite sure about the cerebrospinal fluid pressure; on surgical exposure and on the post mortem table, there were no indications of increased pressure.

It is true that the original concept of otitic hydrocephalus has undergone some modifications (SYMONDS, 1937 and 1944) and, especially, it has been found that ventricular dilatation amounting to internal hydrocephalus need not be present, and, in fact, often is absent in cases which otherwise fall under this descriptive term. In the above case, as in others (WEBER, 1957) the absence of ventricular dilatation does not rule out the diagnosis of otitic "hydrocephalus" if we accept this terminology although there is no conclusive evidence as to the underlying pathology. The subject will be taken up again in the following case history (case M, not included in Table 8).

Case M. Acute otitis media in an infant, aged 2, progressing, despite myringotomy, to bilateral mastoid infection, and rapidly increasing internal hydrocephalus. No response to chemotherapy. Ventricular drainage. No meningitis. No localising signs indicating abscess. Pronounced and enduring decerebrate attitude. Death 34 days after admission. No necropsy allowed.

A 2-year-old native male was admitted with the tentative diagnosis of otogenous meningitis. There was a history of an ear infection 2 weeks before admission, and the left ear was discharging since that time. At the same time a marked retraction of the head and stiffness of all limbs had been noticed. Examination revealed a high temperature and an enlarged and bulging fontanel. There was marked optisthotonus with intense head retraction, and all four limbs were stiff like rigid rods. The head circumference was 19 inches i.e. within normal limits. No convulsions or tonic fits were noticed. X-rays of the skull were normal at that time. Needle exploration through the anterior fontanel was carried out on the right. There was no subdural effusion and the ventricular fluid was clear, containing 12 lymphocytes and 3 polymorphs to the cmm. Both the protein and sugar were 65 mgm per 100 ccm.

Three days after admission a right myringotomy was done; the infant's condition remained unsatisfactory after that and his temperature stayed between 104 and 105° F. Also the head remained retracted and a classical arc de cercle attitude of the torso developed. Both the arms and legs were fully stretched and adducted with the wrists and fingers in flexion. The ankles were fixed in plantar flexion. There was tympanic resonance on percussion over both sides of the head. At a bilateral mastoidotomy cholesteatomatous masses were removed from either side, and the bone showed clear signs of infection. The dura mater and transverse sinus were exposed and appeared normal. The dura was not opened and no needling for an abscess was attempted though, to the E.N.T. specialist, a temporal lobe abscess was a possibility. Under streptomycin, the temperature gradually came down to 99.8° F; however, the decerebrate rigor even became worse and the anterior fontanel remained tense and bulging. An increase of the head circumference by 33 mm. was noticed within 12 days, and the sutures were now clearly separated. Ventricular drainage was instituted. The cannula entered the ventricle 2 cm. beneath skin level. The ventricular fluid was clear and colourless and escaped under considerable pressure. A positive pressure level of 15 cm. was maintained and, after a few days, increased gradually to 20 cm. by elevating the drainage bottle. The fontanel and the widened sutures soon softened down and became subsequently even slightly depressed. Nevertheless, the procedure had no influence on the rigidity which remained unchanged for nearly 5 weeks from the onset up to the patient's death which occurred 9 days after insertion of the ventricular catheter through which, by this time, nearly 1000 ccm. of clear fluid had drained. Ante mortem the temperature climbed again to 105° F. No consent for post mortem examination was obtained.

Comment. Were it not for the unfortunate lack of post mortem evidence this case could well be classified among those commonly (though somewhat loosely) termed otitic hydrocephalus. The prominent clinical features were: sudden onset of hydrocephalic enlargement by the time when the ear infection had reached the mastoid bone; rapid progress despite chemotherapy; absence of meningitis of clinical significance; persistent head retraction and decerebrate attitude (which, however, had been present since the onset of illness), indicating mid-collicular transection, and not relieved by ventricular drainage. Are we right in interpreting the enduring decerebration in terms of an upward cerebellar herniation due to infratentorial abscess or obstruction at the level of the foramen of MAGENDI?

4. The infratentorial group

Case 3.8 may serve to illustrate some of the difficulties and pitfalls in diagnosing an otogenous cerebellar abscess. In cases such as this, with equivocal or conflicting signs,

exploratory burr holes at appropriate sites (Fig. 60) and needling with the brain cannula above and below the transverse sinus are well-advised and, as a rule, either confirm the presence of an abscess or result in establishing an internal hydrocephalus or pyocephalus. A moderate degree of ventricular enlargement is obviously consistent with the diagnosis of subacute purulent meningitis and ventriculitis. In addition, sero-purulent or frankly purulent collections may develop especially at the sites of subarachnoid pools, such as the great cistern or within the cerebello-pontine angle; the latter presumably is identical with what has been termed peduncular or floccular abscess by COURVILLE (1950). It may give rise to unilateral cerebellar signs. The question of tuberculous meningitis not infrequently arises and may remain unsettled, to the naked eye, even on the post mortem table; this is also clearly shown by the case history 3.8 (Table 8).

Concomitant leptomeningeal reaction in either simple mastoid infection or extradural abscess may give rise to pronounced pleocytosis in the

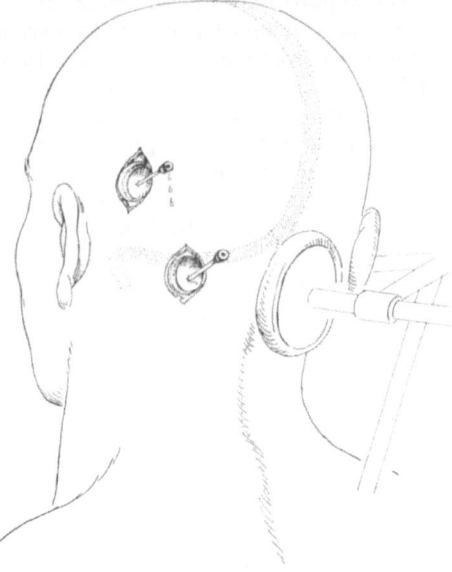

Fig. 60. To show the use of an adjustable head rest in performing exploratory trephine openings at routine sites for needling for an otogenous abscess above and below the tentorium

cerebrospinal fluid. In one of our cases not included here, a cloudy spinal fluid contained 1,300 white cells, and the condition cleared up rapidly after mastoidotomy which had revealed the bone well diseased, but nowhere frank pus.

In cases with suspected abscess in the posterior fossa a spinal tap will rarely be feasible. It is therefore interesting that WEBER (1957) in his cases of chronic cerebellar abscess of otitic origin found a pleocytosis in the lumbar fluid only occasionally, in some instances the cell count was even normal, and associated with increase in protein. The diagnosis of a cerebellar abscess should be reviewed in the presence of a marked increase in the cell count in the cerebrospinal fluid.

The great majority of acute cerebellar abscesses such as suspected during or at the close of a mastoid operation, for obvious reasons will be dealt with by the aural surgeon. The neurosurgeon usually enters the scene only after the ear infection has been brought under control with or without operation. From what has been reported by authors with more extensive experience in this field (SCHREIBER, 1941; FINCHER, 1946; PENNYBACKER, 1948; CHIASSERINI jr., 1960) it becomes evident that, at the stage of chronic cerebellar abscess, unilateral cerebellar signs, especially incoördination of the ipsilateral arm, ataxy and nystagmus, as a rule, are so prominent as to allow the diagnosis without the aid of ancillary procedures. This has recently again been stressed by WEBER (1957) who has treated four cases of chronic cerebellar abscess following otitis media; he also points out that papilloedema is not a common feature. The absence of intracranial pressure signs in cases of cerebellar abscess was earlier mentioned by ERASMUS (1950). PENNYBACKER, in his comprehensive study (1948) based on 18 cerebellar abscesses treated in Oxford, found no papilloedema nor increase in the spinal fluid pressure in several of his patients. In our case 3.9 which is the only instance in the above series of a cerebellar abscess of otitic origin there was a bilateral papilloedema and we abstained from a spinal tap.

A mild 6th nerve weakness was found opposite to the affected ear in this Indian girl, and interpreted to be due to the increased pressure; however, WEBER mentions homolateral paresis of the sixth cranial nerve among localising signs.

The exploring cannula is most likely to encounter an otogenous cerebellar abscess in the lateral and upper parts of the cerebellar hemisphere. Evidently, this is an indication of the most common route of infection viz. through the lateral, triangular part of the cerebellar aspects of the petrous bone.

There is another point of interest both in radical excision of a cerebellar abscess and in instillating into the abscess cavity, solutions of antibiotics and sulpha drugs in higher concentration; it is related, too, to the contiguous spread of infection prevailing in these cases. FINCHER, in dissecting an encapsulated otogenous cerebellar abscess found (to quote him verbatim) "the final dural attachment of the capsule at the petrosal dura". Equally, PENNYBACKER (1948) emphasized this point and conceded that excision of a cerebellar abscess adherent to the petrous bone may require high technical skill to avoid rupture of an otherwise tough capsule. The part of the abscess, facing the petrous bone, therefore, would seem to be a weak spot through which, one would surmise in our case, the instilled solution of concentrated antibiotics leaked out and flooded the cerebrospinal pools around the 4th ventricle followed by a status epilepticus and other serious, yet, in this case, reversible consequences.

5. Tap as against excision

Surgical approach to otogenous cerebellar abscesses mainly centers around the two procedures which have been advocated, at times somewhat dogmatically and to the exclusion of the other, by followers of either method. It would be futile, on the base of a single instance, to take side in the controversy. Nevertheless, a few remarks may not seem out of place.

It has been proved beyond doubt that permanent cure can be achieved by simple tap evacuation; SCHREIBER's series of eight cases is indeed impressive. PENNYBACKER, although he saw complete recovery brought about by decompression and repeated aspiration in two cases (out of eighteen) stated that, as a rule, he feels confident only after removal in toto of a cerebellar abscess. Again, it is obvious from PENNYBACKER's description that radical excision of a cerebellar abscess can be undertaken only with the assistance of a fully equipped neurosurgical unit. On the other hand, tap evacuation will relieve effectively and at once critical pressure levels and, if carried out in time and with a minimum of instrumental and personal assistance, is likely to preclude sudden deaths occurring despite absence of all signs of imminent disaster.

From these considerations it seems reasonable to reserve radical operation for those cases where symptoms continue, despite repeated and, at the end, negative aspirations, and thorotrast or air pyograms reveal the abscess failing to dry up. Evidently, solid granulomas such as described by WEBER (1957) and the one discussed in Chapter E (case 5.3) call a limine for removal by standard craniotomy.

6. Traumatic cases

There is little to comment on the four traumatic cases listed above under 3.10 to 3.13. The time of onset of intradural suppuration following skull fractures in the vicinity of the petrous bone is of interest and may vary considerably. In case 3.10 who had an open fracture of the mastoid region, clinical signs of intradural infection developed only four weeks after injury; by this time, a discharging sinus in the scalp had formed. In the presence of concealed damage to the bone not revealed on routine X-rays signs of meningitis may be manifest as early as the 3rd day; a typical instance is case 3.12. Thus, the infection may spread by contiguity from the infected mastoid cells (as in case 3.10), or the subarachnoid spaces may be directly opened up by the injury (as in case 3.12) giving rise to a meningitis of the type which was called "meningitis of very early onset" by CAIRNS and assoc. (1947) and which has been discussed earlier (p. 31). In case 3.13 the indication for operation of a profuse traumatic otorrhoea persisting for ten days can hardly be doubted, and was suggested by the positive X-ray findings and the presence of an intracranial aerocele, a potential precursor of meningitis, even in the chemotherapeutic era.

It is true that following BUCY's argument (1938) in case of dural leak, conservative handling of the patient would have been a possible alternative. BUCY, from own experiences with invariably good results in six patients, advocated the TRENDELENBURG tilt and forcing fluids in order to maintain free escape of the cerebrospinal fluid, instead of flooding, by lumbar taps, the cerebrospinal fluid pathways with potentially infected material.

The extradural approach along the floor of the middle fossa such as performed in case 3.13 met with the two pitfalls likely to occur in such cases viz. a brisk bleed from the middle meningeal artery, and damage to the facial nerve, possibly due to extensive cauterization of the superior petrosal sinus; in our patient the facial weakness still persisted at the time of his discharge from the hospital.

The immediate post-operative result in this man was disappointing, the dural leak continued, and nothing was achieved by continuous spinal drainage; the draining catheter soon clogged whereupon the patient improved promptly and the cerebrospinal fluid leak subsided; so, eventually, the operation was successful.

The early type of brain abscess following a missile wound in case 3.11 behaved as far as we know, precisely in the same way as early abscesses on the convexity discussed in Chapter B; there was no dural leak and no hemiparesis; the aphasia improved promptly after wound toilet and drainage of the abscess.

D. Metastatic brain abscesses

1. Etiology and pathogenesis

In Table 9 the eight cases included in this series are summarized together with a short survey of the neurological and operative findings. There were two recoveries, three operative deaths, one patient died on her way to the hospital. In two cases the outcome is unkown.

Blood-borne infections of the brain reach the central nervous system from various distant sources. Among the eight metastatic brain abscesses to be discussed here, three were classified as thoracogenic. In case 4.8 the chest lesion was on the same side as the brain abscess; in case 4.6 the lesions were on opposite sides; in case 4.1 the side of broncho-pneumonia was not stated.

It is worth mentioning that, with regard to the pulmonary lesion, the radiologist only in one case considered bronchiectasis a possibility such as concealed behind a consolida-tion of two lobes. Also in case 4.8 bronchiectasis was possible (Fig. 61); there was no time

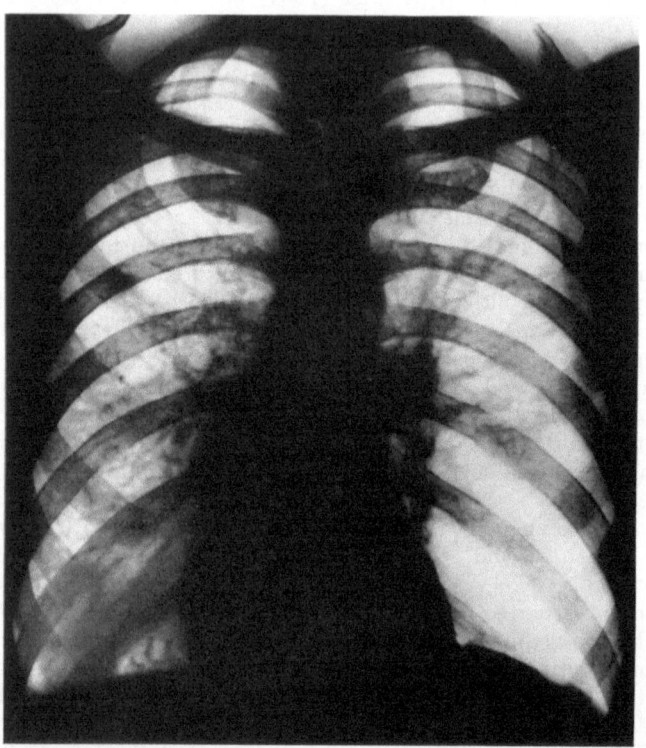

Fig. 61. Radiological appearance of chest in a man, aged 30, who, according to history obtained, had collapsed at work and slipped into a semicoma associated with left hemiplegia. He had bilateral papilloedema. A rönt-genogram of his chest revealed consolidation of the right lower lobe and a possible, partial, pneumothorax on left. (There was a vague history of recent injury to his chest.) Angiography (see following Fig. 62) disclosed a thoracogenic abscess in the right cerebral hemisphere. (Case 4.8)

to confirm this by bronchography and the postoperative course in this patient hardly lends support to this view. It is of interest to note that earlier writers have stated that bronchiectasis was the chief cause of metastatic brain abscesses. (The SCHORSTEIN Lecture on abscess of the brain 1909). In contrast to this view, GOWERS[1] held empyema to be the most common pulmonary antecedent of brain abscesses.

A further point deserves mentioning here. In the SCHORSTEIN Lecture, just mentioned, a series of 18 thoracogenic brain abscesses were presented; the left hemisphere was found more often affected than the right. This view is shared, apparently on post mortem obser-vations, by PETERS (1951), among others. It has been thought that the arterial route from the left heart via the left carotid artery being more straightforward than on the right accounts for the preferential involvement of the left hemisphere in blood-borne metastases

---

[1] Diseases of the Brain, 1888.

Table 9. *Synopsis, clinical and pathological, of 8 cases of blood-borne abscess of the brain*

Case no. (age)	Clinical	Site of abscess	Operation	Outcome
4.1 (adult)	Bronchopneumonia about 4 weeks previously	Left temporal	Aspiration and drainage (iodoform wick) as an emergency measure	Died shortly after operation
4.2 (39)	Short-lived history of raised intracranial pressure; sedimentation rate increased; X-rays of chest normal. Brain abscess suspected; arteriography disclosed avascularity in right hemisphere	Right postero-parietal (para-sagittal)	Exploratory trephine and needling; thick foul pus encountered 2 cm. from surface; osteoplastic craniotomy, decapping and radical excision; thin capsule ruptured	Unknown
4.3 (20)	Pyelonephritis one year previously, followed by "rheumatoid" pain; recently severe headache; high papilloedema with retinal haemorrhages. Homonymous hemianopia to right, questionable facial weakness on right; sedimentation rate markedly increased	Left occipital	Exploring cannula meets resistance 1—2 cms. from surface; aspiration of 15 ml. of thick yellow pus; culture negative. Left occipital lobectomy including abscess with thick capsule (Fig. 63)	Unknown
4.4 (adult)	Tonsilectomy 6 weeks previously. Neck glands on right and right jugular vein became thickened and tender. 4 weeks after onset sudden left hemiparesis and mixed type of aphasia developed, with septicaemia and left jacksonian fits. No papilloedema	Tonsillo-genous multiple abscesses throughout right hemisphere	After evacuation of subdural abscess overlying right temporal and rolandic areas, temperature remained high and signs of meningitis developed	Died 11 days after subdural tap. Necropsy: 4 brain abscesses in right hemisphere; purulent meningitis and thrombophlebitis extending into dural sinuses on both sides. Muco-purulent otitis media on right. Multiple small abscesses in left lung, with fresh pleuresy
4.5 (32)	Apoplectic onset with hemiplegia and coma, 8 days before death (1944)	Right parietal	Died on her way to the hospital	Necropsy:[1] Multiple abscesses in right parietal lobe; spreading oedema and suppurative encephalitis. Signs of acute rise in intracranial pressure; neurogenous haemorrhages in both lungs
4.6 (± 60)	No history available (Native). Admitted in stupor and excessive emaciation; halitosis suggesting pulmonary gangraen. No papilloedema. Aphasia. Hemiparesis on right. X-rays of chest: Consolidation of right middle and lower lobes, with possible bronchiectases. Carotid angiography: elevation of left sylvian group	Left temporo-parietal	Exploratory burr hole in either parietal region made; 10 ml. of clear fluid aspirated from right ventricle 2 inch. from surface. 25 ml. of flocculent, offensive, pus aspirated from left hemisphere and replaced by air and a solution of 20,000 u of penicillin	Air over both hemispheres and alongside falx cerebri on left; right ventricle small, hardly displaced. Pat. died the following day. No autopsy allowed. Bacteriology: pus from abscess yielded non-haemolytic streptococci; fluid from right ventricle: no growth
4.7 (12)	About 1 weeks' history of headache, stiff neck and mental dullness. Lumbar fluid: 50 polymorphs and lymphocytes. Air instilled and went up to stop at the tentorium level. Increasing drowsiness. Admitted in great pain, with normal temperature; possible aphasia (African native); field defect to right. Left angiography: expanding avascular lesion outlined	Left parieto-occipital	Left parietal burr hole made, dura slack. Abscess struck 2 inch. from surface and 30 ml. of thick stinking pus aspirated; cavity washed with saline; thick rubber catheter inserted. Systemic and local penicillin through catheter; had one epileptic convulsion. Pus: g + cocci and bacilli. No growth. On right: clear fluid from ventricle aspirated	Slow recovery. Drain removed after 10 days, wound healed p.pr. Discharged 5$^1/_2$ weeks after evacuation of abscess; slight weakness of right arm; no gross field defect. Scalp over trephine indrawn and pulsating

[1] Performed by Professor R. RÖSSLE.

Table 9. (Continued)

Case no. (age)	Clinicial	Site of abscess	Operation	Outcome
4.8 (30)	Conflicting history (African native): Epilepsy? Collapsed at work following injury to his chest and slipped into semicoma with left hemiplegia. Bilateral papilloedema. No temperature. Lumbar fluid: 4 lymphocytes, protein slightly elevated. X-rays of chest: consolidation of right lower lobe (Fig. 61). Right carotid angiography: expanding mass in posterior frontal region; paucity of blood supply indicating cyst or abscess (Fig. 62)	Right frontal (posterior part)	Right fronto-temporal osteoplastic flap; dura slack, brain soft, "fluctuating". Cannula entered an abscess cavity from which 20 ml. of discoloured, stinking, flocculent, pus mixed with debris was aspirated, cavity refilled with mixture of antibiotics, cannula replaced by rubber catheter, dura re-sutured, wound closed in layers	Quick recovery, daily instillations of antibiotics; catheter removed after 7 days, wound healed p.pr. Discharged 5 weeks after operation with slight left facial weakness, chest X-rays normal. Re-admitted 8 weeks later with fits and a subaponeurotic "bag" of pus which was incised and drained. Air studies were normal at that time. Discharged with scalp wound closed

of any sort. It seems doubtful, however, whether the anatomical configuration of the arch of the aorta and its main branches supports such view. Alternatively, it would seem likely that the avenue to the brain is gained by emboli from the chest by way of the vertebral veins as suggested by COLLIS thus accounting for the fact that in some series like the one of RIZZOLI et al. the side of the cerebral lesion corresponded to the side of pulmonary pathology.

In case 4.4 of the above series a twofold etiology appears to be a possibility; septic thrombophlebitis of the right internal jugular vein together with septicaemia followed a tonsilectomy, and, in turn, was followed, within four weeks, by localizing cerebral signs leading eventually to evacuation of a subdural empyema. Eleven days later, the patient died with signs of diffuse purulent meningitis. Autopsy then revealed, in addition to multiple brain abscesses, a muco-purulent otitis media. Both, the ear infection and the brain abscesses were on the same side as the previous jugular phlebitis.

In 2 cases in our series the primary source of infection remained obscure clinically; in one patient who did not even reach the operating theatre post mortem examination by Professor R. RÖSSLE provided no clue as to the primary nidus of infection. In case 4.3 a pyelonephritis was a possible cause of the brain abscess preceding its clinical signs by one year.

The acute onset and rapid progress of cerebral involvement in case 4.8, together with the radiological findings in the chest, at first sight suggested interpretation in terms of cerebral embolism. Cases of so-called "hemiplégie pneumique et pleurétique" have been described by French authors and again mentioned by HILLER in his classical contribution to the Handbuch der Neurologie (1936).

2. Carotid angiography

In the case just mentioned as in three others carotid *angiography* was an important diagnostic procedure confirming, in every case, type and site of the suspected lesion (Fig. 62).

This applies equally to brain abscesses in general whatever their etiology as pointed out in a recent paper by BALLANTINE and SHEALY[1].

In this respect, case 4.6 deserves special comment. The arteriogram here disclosed local displacement of the sylvian group in line with an expanding lesion in the temporal lobe, but negligible shift of the anterior cerebral across the midline; lack of any degree of midline displacement was confirmed by air studies. A bilateral abscess was ruled out by contralateral angiography as well as by ventricular tap on the side opposite the abscess;

---

[1] The reader is referred to the recent paper by G. WEBER: L'angiographie dans le diagnostic des abscès cérébraux. Neuro-Chirurgie **6**, 317 (1960).

yet, there were unequivocal signs of tentorial coning such as lowered level of consciousness and oculomotor paresis on the side of the abscess. There was no papilloedema and, in keeping with this, no signs of increased pressure were found beneath the bilateral trephine openings; the brain surface was pulsating in a normal fashion. It would seem, thus, that break-down and liquefaction of cerebral tissue within the hemisphere involved, in this case, had taken place pari passu with accumulation of pus to such extent as to outweigh the mass of the growing abscess. This view is corroborated by the presence of necrotic tissue and debris aspirated from the abscess cavity.

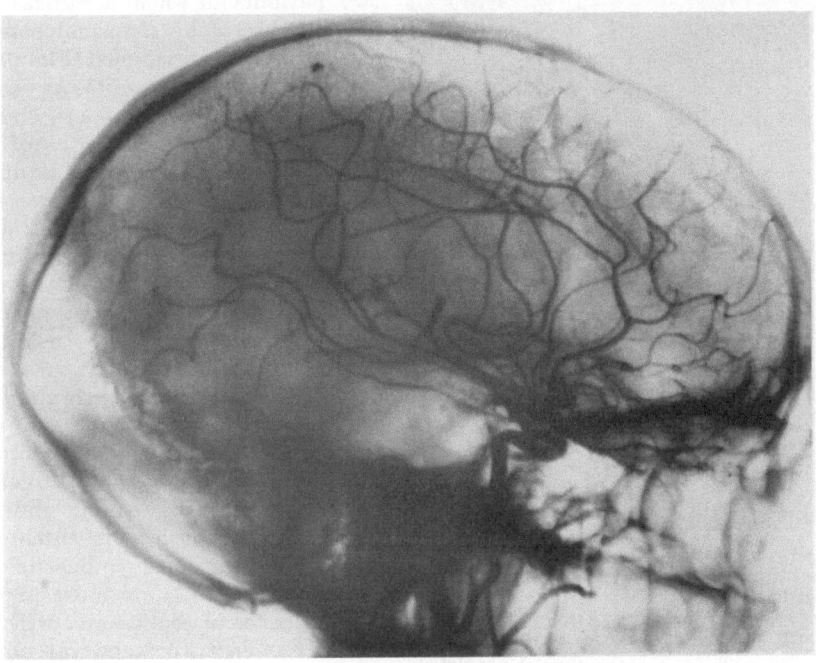

Fig. 62. Carotid angiogram (lateral view) in a case of thoracogenic brain abscess in right hemisphere. The a.-p. view shews flattening of the bifurcation of the internal carotid artery and marked shift across the midline. On the lateral view the ascendent branches of the sylvian group are streched and splayed out indicating an expanding mass in posterior part of frontal lobe. Subsequently, the abscess was tapped and aspirated. The patient recovered. (Case 4.8)
NB. Compare with angiogram in patient with intracerebral clot at same site, shown in Fig. 6

In addition, this patient may be taken as another instance of a cerebral abscess beneath a healthy looking and pulsatile dura mater; it is not the only one in the series; also in cases 4.7 and 4.8 the dura was conspicuously slack and the abscess cavity in patient 4.8 again contained flocculent pus mixed with debris.

Similar experiences have been made by some aural surgeons in cases of otogenous temporal lobe abscess as shown conclusively by ATKINSON who rightly pointed out that an apparently normal and pulsating dura mater must by no means be taken as evidence against an underlying brain abscess.

3. Surgical intervention

Turning now to the problems of surgical intervention it will be seen from Table 9 that simple aspiration and drainage was done in four i.e. half of the cases and of these two patients died shortly after the procedure, though in case 4.6 it should be conceded that pulmonary gangraen and advanced emaciation were both important factors contributing to the fatal outcome. Cases 4.7 and 4.8 both recovered after evacuation and drainage under adequate systemic and local chemotherapy; the latter was carried out through the drain which was removed after 10 and 7 days respectively. It must be realized, however, that the follow-up period in both cases which was 5$^1/_2$ weeks and 10 weeks respectively, if far too short to allow final assessment; especially in case 4.8 some doubt will arise regarding a lasting cure in view of the patient's re-admission because of local suppuration underneath the scalp at the site of previous drainage which necessitated surgical evacuation. In addition, this patient was reported to have convulsions which possibly heralded an extradural or even intradural extension although this was not evidenced by air studies during his second stay in hospital. In the two patients in whom a radical excision of the abscess by a formal osteoplastic craniotomy was performed (Fig. 63) unfortunately no follow-up notes are available.

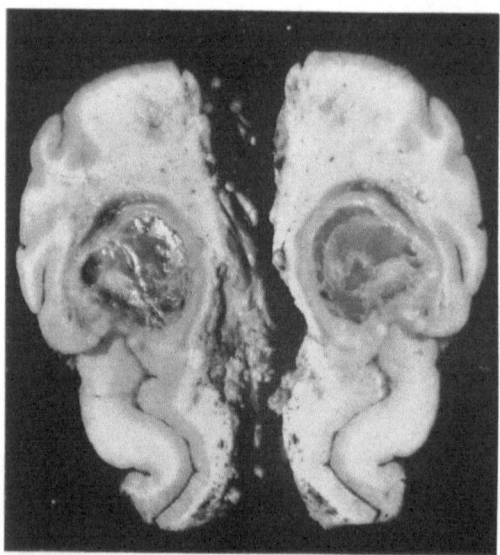

Fig. 63. Operative specimen from a girl aged 20 years, with a metastatic abscess in left occipital lobe. She had high papilloedema with retinal haemorrhages and an homonymous hemanopia to the right. Occipital lobectomy was performed including the abscess surrounded by a thick membrane. Culture from the abscess was sterile. (Case 4.3, 1943)

The importance of modern chemotherapy is stressed by the series of RIZZOLI et al. Their group of ten metastatic brain abscesses, seven of which were thoracogenic, were treated between 1942 and 1946 by various surgeons and all patients were cured; one case recovered without operation. All patients had chemotherapy either before or after surgery or both, mostly penicillin and sulfadiazine. It is a common experience that metastatic brain abscesses may present as true emergencies i.e. with symptoms and signs of pressure cone which, in these instances, may well overshadow any localizing signs; among these, some sort of aphasia such as in cases 4.4, 4.6, and 4.7, and a homonymous field defect (cases 4.3 and 4.7) are most prominent. The presence of septicaemia with blood-borne meningitis or subdural empyema, as well as a debilitating condition of long standing such as bronchiectasis or pulmonary gangraen will not permit unduly long expectant treatment but will call for some kind of surgery be it a single trephine opening and aspiration. It is in these cases where modern full-range chemotherapy plays its important part; this is clearly shown by the cases 4.7 and 4.8 in contrast to case 4.4 in which chemotherapy, such as was available in 1941, failed to control the slow but definite spread from a local nidus of infection via a regional thrombophlebitis to septicaemia with multiple pyaemic metastases. It is an open question whether such development from local to generalized infection can now be safely prevented by means of chemotherapy. In the above series a comparison of the cases treated before 1944 with those after 1956, reflects clearly the advances in chemotherapy brought about during the last fifteen years.

E. Fungal infections*

Brain abscesses due to saprophytic fungi, such as moulds and yeasts, are uncommon; consequently, single cases and small series of two and three cases are still held worth while describing.

* The reader is referred to the article „Die tierischen Parasiten und Pilzinfektionen im zentralen Nervensystem" by MATTOS-PIMENTA, A., and P. BRANDT, in Handbuch der Neurochirurgie, herausgegeben von H. OLIVECRONA u. W. TÖNNIS, Bd. IV/1. Berlin: Springer 1960.

In 1949, Craig and Gates from the Mayo Foundation, have found five "mycotic" abscesses among a series of 105 metastatic brain abscesses; the authors express their doubt as to what appears to them a low incidence of 4.8% and they point out that one third of their cultures yielded a negative result probably due to intensive chemotherapy or the presence of fungi as causative agents. The fungi established in the 5 cases of Craig and Gates, were: Candida (Monilia) albicans in one, Coccidioides and Actinomyces (to which the species Nocardia belongs), each in two patients. One of the abscesses due to coccidiosis was in the left cerebellar hemisphere and the patient died after drainage and despite chemotherapy. False localizing signs were present, caused by a localized hygroma between the arachnoid and pia, in a patient with a right frontal abscess due to C. albicans.

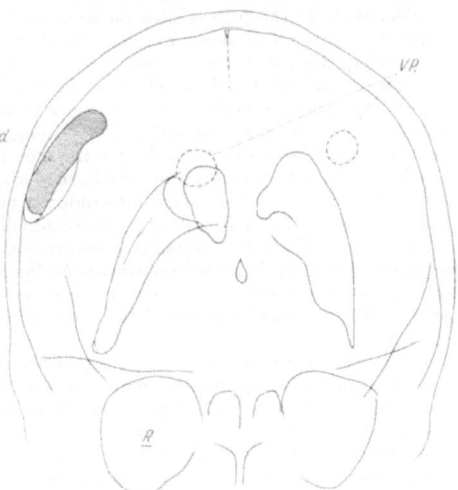

Three cases seen by the present writer during recent years in South Africa will be reported here in some detail. One is a cerebral nocardiosis following a penetrating trauma to the head; one is a blastomycotic abscess in the occipital lobe; and the last one is a rare case of tumour-like torulosis of the cerebellum.

Case 5.1. Fistulous cerebral nocardiosis following penetrating injury one year previously. Low grade meningitis. Moderate ventricular dilatation. Death from intraventricular haemorrhage following excision of scarred mass with scattered abscesses.

This adult Bantu male was admitted with the diagnosis of traumatic late brain abscess following penetrating injury to the right fronto-parietal region. He had been hit with a blunt instrument one year previously, and had bled from his nose. He related that he was knocked unconscious for about an hour. Two weeks after the incident a weakness of his left arm and leg was noticed and he was then admitted to a district hospital with a purulent discharging sinus over the right pre-motor area. It was also reported that somewhat later "an abscess had been opened at this site".

Fig. 64. Ventriculogram (p.-a. view) in a case of cerebral nocardiosis following penetrating injury. Note defect in bone (d) on right, moderate enlargement of both lateral ventricles, and absence of gross shift as well as local extension of right ventricle to the defect in the vault (Case 5.1) VP marks burr holes

On admission he was found to have a pulsating, in-drawn, defect in the vault, 2 by 2¹/₂ inches in size, in the region of the right coronal suture. There was some scarring of the scalp in this area and two sinuses discharging thick creamy-coloured pus were present. Mentally he was slow but responsive. The optic discs were normal and so were the ocular movements. There was a hemiparesis of the left arm and face. X-rays of the skull revealed a roundish, smooth-edged, defect in the skull at the above region. No in-driven fragments or foreign bodies were present. A lumbar tap shewed a pressure of 150 mms. with normal dynamics on Queckenstedt's test. The fluid was hazy, with a yellowish tinge. About 75 ml. of the fluid were then replaced by air. On subsequent X-rays only the subarachnoid spaces between the two hemispheres and within the sylvian fossae were visualized, no air had entered the ventricles. There was no indication of a shift across the midline or of gross distortion of the parts filled with air. The lumbar fluid was reported to contain: ++ polymorphonuclears, + lymphocytes. No organisms were found and the culture was negative. Five days after the lumbar air studies a ventriculography was performed through posteroparietal burr holes. There were no signs of raised pressure on the dura and the brain surface; both were pulsating nicely. The ventricular fluid was hazy and colourless; about one fluid ounce was replaced by air. X-rays disclosed moderate dilatation of the lateral ventricles, the left ventricle being slightly more involved than the right one. The contours of the left ventricle were somewhat rounded off whereas on the right, corresponding to the site of the skull defect, the roof of the lateral ventricle shewed slight distortion and depression. There was no shift of the septum pellucidum, the slit-like 3rd ventricle, or the aqueduct. Both temporal horns were visualized by air, they were comparatively large and not displaced. On the lateral face-up view, there was a crescent-shaped subdural air deposit overlying one of the frontal poles (Fig. 64).

Despite combined treatment with penicillin and chloramphenicol the patient failed to improve, and the discharge from the scalp sinuses continued. It was therefore decided to operate and to follow up the sinuses as deep as possible in an attempt to excise them together with the surrounding scar tissue. The operation was carried out under local anaesthesia one week following ventriculography.

7*

From a trefoliate incision encompassing the sinus openings the scalp was reflected and a solid deep-rooted scar was exposed involving the dura and the brain alike; it contained numerous tracks and small abscesses all filled with thick, intensely yellow pus; following down one of the tracks into the depth a bigger abscess was entered and its contents removed by suction; this was followed by a gush of cerebrospinal fluid from the adjacent ventricle. The dense fibrotic capsule was now excised carefully and without any more ventricular leak. A smooth-walled cavity resulted, about 7 cms. deep as measured from the surface. A doubled-up soft rubber drain was issued through the wound.

The patient succumbed suddenly the following day. Autopsy revealed fresh blood filling the ventricular system. No brain abscess or purulent meningitis was present to the naked eye. Examination of the pus from the abscess revealed gram + mycelial threads which were identified as being of the genus *Nocardia* (Pathological Institute of the Pretoria University).

Comment. In this patient intracranial suppuration was due to infection by a fungus of the genus nocardia. Evidence of this was obtained from the pus of one of the multiple abscesses during craniotomy. Unfortunately, the purulent discharge from the sinus on the scalp was not examined bacteriologically.

Intracranial infection followed a penetrating trauma to the skull in the right fronto-parietal region which the patient had suffered about one year prior to admission leaving him with a bony defect which subsequently was surgically enlarged, and with a discharging sinus at the site of trauma. After surgical intervention and local drainage of an abscess (according to the report obtained), the discharge nevertheless continued, at intervals, and, as time went on, multiple sinuses formed surrounded by an area of scarring overlying the surgical defect in the vault. The discharge was creamy-coloured, non-offensive pus; obviously, this was the reason for suspecting a brain abscess and bringing the patient eventually under neurosurgical care.

Yet, signs of raised intracranial pressure were absent, as far as we know, throughout. The soft tissues overlying the skull defect were in-drawn and pulsatile. The optic discs were sharply outlined and of normal colour; mental dullness as exhibited by this Bantu male probably was due, in part, to his chronic meningitis which will be discussed presently. The ventriculogram gave no indication of a space-occupying mass of surgical proportions.

The absence of raised pressure in spite of several deep-seated brain abscesses (though they were of moderate size) calls for some explanation; there was a solid block of mesodermal scar surrounding and separating the abscesses and replacing the nervous tissue, with its well-known tendency to shrinking; even so, it is remarkable that no diverticulum-like extension of the lateral ventricle corresponding to the defect in the bone, was disclosed on the ventriculogram (Fig. 64). Furthermore, the presence of air within the subarachnoid and subdural spaces indicated moderate generalized atrophy of the nervous tissue.

The chronic meningitis as evidenced by the lumbar fluid is somewhat difficult to account for. No organisms were cultured from the fluid. Was it a primary invasion of the subarachnoid pathways due to the penetrating injury one year previously? Initial involvement and infection of the ventricle by the trauma is a possibility since details regarding the injury are lacking. Could a fungal infection of the subarachnoid spaces linger on for months in a dormant, subclinical fashion? On surgical exposure, one of the abscesses was very close to, but not communicating with the lateral ventricle; it seems plausible that this accounted for the pleocytosis in the lumbar fluid.

Finally, to account for the fatal outcome which clearly was due to intraventricular haemorrhage, it should be remembered that in an attempt to en-block resection of that scar containing a veritable maze of tracks with scattered small abscesses, confluent in the depth, to form bigger cavities, it was exceptionally difficult to follow the individual tracks; they were tethered to the dura mater as well as to the ventricular wall; in fact, this scar had formed during a long course of lingering suppuration inside and outside the skull; this made haemostasis a delicate and precarious procedure.

Case 5.2. Blastomycotic abscess in the right occipitoparietal area. Short history. Rapid progress with signs of high intracranial pressure; no signs of meningitis. Sudden death 16 days after evacuation and drainage.

A Bantu male, aged 23, was admitted with a history of bitemporal headache and dizziness which had developed 10 days before admission. He had vomited once. On examination he was groaning with pain, pointing to the right side of his head, and slightly dazed but co-operative. There was bilateral papilloedema. The left pupil was slightly larger and its reaction to light somewhat sluggish as compared to the right. There was a doubtful 6th nerve paresis on the left. No nystagmus was present. An homonymous hemianopia had already been found by the referring doctor and confirmed on the ward. On special questioning the patient admitted that he had been unable to see properly things on his left side one month prior to the onset of his headache. There was weakness of his left arm and leg; the deep reflexes were equal but both knee reflexes were absent. A key put into his left palm was identified, with closed eyes, as an "object made of iron". Radiology of his skull revealed no signs of raised pressure nor any abnormal calcarious deposits. On lumbar puncture, the fluid was under considerable pressure; two polymorphonuclears per cmm. were reported, and the proteins were "slightly raised". The pulse rate was 44 and the blood pressure 130 mm Hg. systolic.

Bilateral burr holes were carried out in the posteroparietal region under local anaesthesia for ventriculography. The dura mater was under excessive pressure on either side and so was the brain on the right side. The brain cannula only after several attempts entered a slit-like ventricle on the right containing a few ml. of clear fluid. On the left, the ventricle was struck at once at a depth of 4 cms. Air replacement was done through ventricular catheters on either side; the catheters were tied off and anchored to the galea. Subsequent X-rays shewed gross displacement beneath the falx to the left. The right occipital horn was pushed forward rather than "amputated" and there was a questionable tumour contouring into the right temporal horn. It was open to debate whether we were dealing with an extracerebral expanding mass in the right occipital region or whether the local indentation into the right inferior horn meant an intracerebral mass (Fig. 65).

Following ventriculography an osteoplastic flap was turned down under local anaesthesia with the patient in the supine position, exposing the greater part of the right occipital and parietal lobes. The catheter from the right ventricle was withdrawn while on the left it remained in situ and was cut short to let fluid escape. The dura was under very high pressure indeed, thinned out and, as it were, translucent so as to permit discernment of a normal pattern of gyri and whitish sulci underneath. The impression was that of a huge subcortical cyst. A cannula was then inserted through the closed dura; it met with but slight resistance and at once turbid

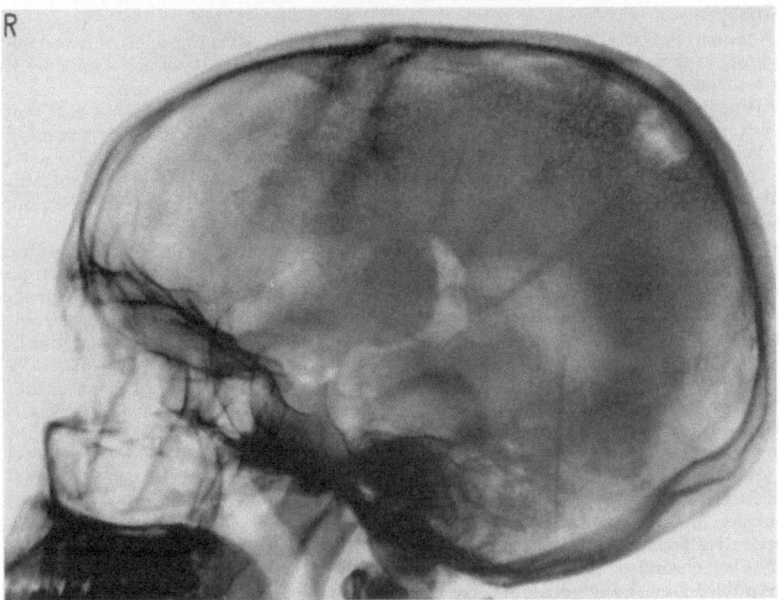

Fig. 65. Ventriculogram (p.-a. lateral view) in a case of blastomycotic abscess in right occipital lobe. Air replacement was done through ventricular catheters. Note gross forward displacement of right occipital horn and tumour contouring in right temporal horn. The patient had been admitted with a short history of rapidly rising intracranial pressure. Note ventricular catheters in situ. (Case 5.2)

fluid escaped from its tip. Aspiration yielded some 30 ml. of greyish-brown, thick, mucoid, pus with a peculiar, not actually offensive smell. Further needling in several directions failed to impart the impression of a multilocular abscess. Radical excision was considered at first but not attempted in view of the thinness of the capsule; in fact, purulent cerebritis with central liquefaction would have been a better term to describe the presenting lesion. So the brain cannula was replaced by a soft rubber catheter and a mixture of penicillin, streptomycin and chloramphenicol was instilled into the cavity, onto the dura which had been contaminated with pus, and into the wound itself. The catheter was issued through one of the burr holes and secured to the periosteum. The bone flap was re-inserted, without using wire, and the flap re-sutured. The patient stood the procedure well; he had received one pint of concentrated plasma.

Intracerebral instillations were continued through the following days and sulphonamides were added for systemic administration. The intracranial pressure was controlled by allowing fluid to escape through the catheter in the left ventricle. On the 3rd day after the operation the patient fell out of his bed and had to be taken to the theatre where, under local anaesthesia, a fresh haematoma from beneath the skin flap was removed; the flap was carefully resutured in 2 layers. Within 6 days following operation the catheter was removed from the abscess and systemic chemotherapy continued. The wound healing was per primary union. There were, by this time, no signs of unilateral weakness but the hemianopia persisted. The patient's general condition remained excellent. On the 16th day following craniotomy the man suddenly went into a deep coma with stertorous breathing at a rate of 6 per min., a feeble pulse and a blood pressure up to 200 mms. Hg. All limbs were flaccid, all voluntary movements absent. Approximately 15 ml. of thick pus were immediately aspirated from the abscess cavity; the patient expired on his way to the theatre.

Post mortem examination revealed a huge fungal abscess occupying the greater parts of the right occipital and parietal lobes; these parts, to the naked eye, resembled a big area of vascular softening rather than a walled-off abscess, there being no proper encapsulation but frank pus inside. Histologically, the lesion was found to consist of granulomatous tissue with numerous giant cells, foci of suppuration, and a large number of pigmented fungal hyphae inside and outside the cells, most likely chromoblastomycetes (Dr. J. van Dyk). The hilar glands in the right lung were caseous but no tuberculous foci were disclosed elsewhere in the body.

Comment. In contrast to the preceding case this was a fungal infection reaching the brain via the blood stream; consequently, no trauma to or infection in the scalp was present here. There were no indications of a primary lesion elsewhere, clinically or on the post mortem table.

No detailed classification of the causal genus was provided by the laboratory but there was much in favour of a chromoblastomycotic type of fungus. From the laboratory where the above case was examined, a metastatic brain abscess due to blastomycetes infection had been reported by Watson and Lines in 1957; their patient apparently was the 3rd case on record, the previous two being reported by Binford et al. (1952) and King et al. (1952) respectively.

The above patient presented with a short-lived history of rapidly advancing signs of raised supratentorial pressure clouding, to some extent, the localizing signs which, nevertheless, were found on close examination so as to allow a diagnosis of the site of the lesion.

A lumbar tap, judiciously carried out revealed, as one would expect, a high pressure and only two polymorphs per cmm. In keeping with this was the absence of clinical signs of meningitis. This is in marked contrast to the case of Watson and Lines already referred to.

Both, on the operating and the autopsy table, the lesion gave the impression of a spreading purulent cerebritis without definite walling-off; on operative exposure, this was the reason for abstaining from an attempt to radical excision.

Obviously, aspiration and drainage for a rather short period of time, as carried out in this case, were only temporary measures for lowering intracranial tension. Chemotherapy, both local and systemic, possibly were helpful in controlling the virulence of the infection but were inadequate in preventing recurrence of raised pressure with consequent fatal coning as soon as the draining catheter had been withdrawn from the abscess cavity. From a case reported by Weber in 1957, it would appear that fungal infection of the human brain may well respond to antibiotics; Weber's patient had a metastatic actinomycotic brain abscess which, on excision, was surrounded by a thick capsule. From the pus anaerobic actinomyces israeli was cultured sensitive, in vitro, to penicillin and streptomycin. The patient, after a dramatic postoperative course, eventually recovered.

It is of some interest to note that the initial anatomical diagnosis in our case was that of tuberculoma of the brain with secondary abscess formation from hilar pulmonary glands. The true nature of the lesion became evident only under the microscope. This confirms a common experience indicating that differential diagnosis of a suspected fungal infection of the central nervous system from tuberculosis often is a clinical as well as an anatomical puzzle. In the above patient a tuberculoma was not considered clinically in view of the short history and operative findings. Also, the absence of meningitis both before and after the operation suggested the absence of tuberculosis. It is the more remarkable that, on the post mortem table, the lesion, at first sight, should have resembled so much a tuberculoma. The point will be raised again in commenting on the following case.

Case 5.3. Tumour-forming cerebellar torulosis in an Indian male who was admitted with symptoms and signs of rapidly increasing intracranial pressure and tonsillar coning. No clinical signs of meningitis. Removal of the granuloma in toto to the naked eye. Recurrence within 7 months. No obstruction of the cerebrospinal fluid-passages though marked ventricular dilatation on lumbar air studies. Considerable improvement on conservative treatment.

An Indian male, aged 19, was admitted to the King Edward VIII Hospital in Durban with a history of headache, dimness of vision, and intermittent vomiting. It was difficult to ascertain details of his history. His headache possibly dated back for 4 months or even 2 years; there was also pain and stiffness at the back of his neck and, for some time, he had been losing weight. His doctor referred him with a tentative diagnosis of tuberculous meningitis. On examination, he was somewhat lethargic and slightly confused. There was a doubtful left facial weakness and definite left ear deafness. He had high papilloedema with patchy haemorrhages on both sides, left-sided cerebellar and right-sided pyramidal signs, the latter being interpreted in terms of cerebellar coning. Lumbar tap, cautiously performed, yielded a fluid containing 100 mg.-% of protein with increased globulins, and no cells. Vertebralis angiography by the femoral route was skillfully carried out by Dr. Brink and revealed gross upward displacement both of the superior cerebellar and posterior cerebral groups thus confirming the diagnosis of an expanding mass in the left half of the posterior fossa. A tentorium meningioma was considered a possibility and thought to extend both sides of the lateral sinus into the supratentorial as well as infratentorial compartments.

Under general anaesthesia and with the patient in the face-down position exposure of the posterior fossa was carried out from a crossbow incision. The posterior arch of the atlas and the occipital squama over both cerebellar hemispheres were taken away. On the left, the dura mater was found bulging and under excessive tension; it appeared as if thinned out. After its incision down to the foramen of Magendi a tongue-like tonsillar herniation came into sight on the left thus confirming the clinical diagnosis. The pia-arachnoid was nicked and cerebrospinal fluid allowed to escape with subsequent relief of pressure. When a brain cannula was inserted through the closed dura over the left cerebellum it struck a hard resistance, too hard, in fact, for an abscess. The dura was now opened and reflected. A surfacing tumour was exposed occupying the greater part of the left compartment, compressing and displacing the left cerebellar hemisphere in a forward and upward direction without actually infiltrating the brain tissue. The tumour extended right up to the tentorium. It was lobulated and, at places, of a conspicuous yellow tinge, and brawny gelatinous appearance. It was thought likely to be

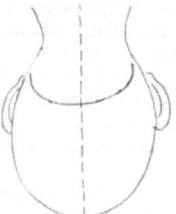

Fig. 66 a

Fig. 66. Exposure of posterior fossa in case of tumour-forming torulosis of left cerebellar hemisphere. Posterior arch of atlas nibbled away and dura mater reflected over the left side to show smooth capsule covering the granuloma, and tongue-like extension of left cerebellar tonsil to form a Cushing's pressure cone. (Case 5.3)

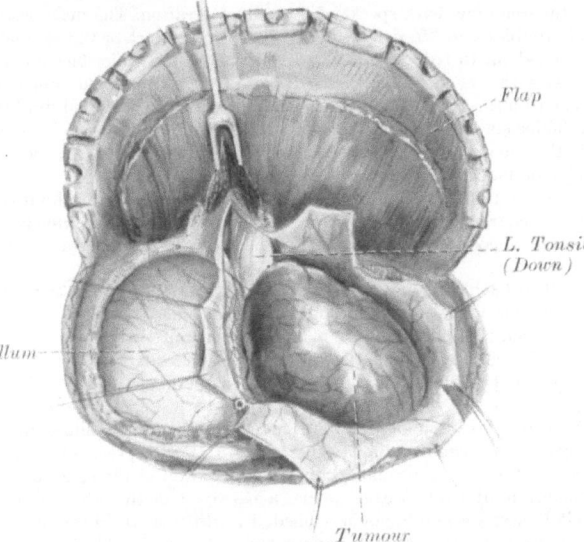

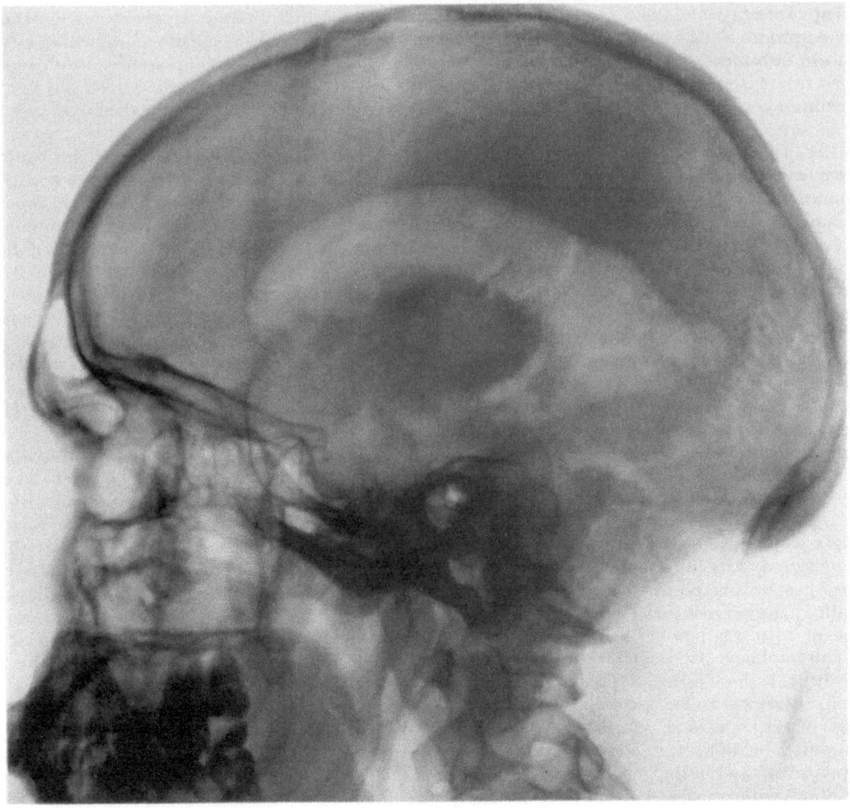

Fig. 66 b

Fig. 67. Lumbar air encephalogram (lateral view) in a case of recurrent tumour-forming cerebellar torulosis. Note ventricular dilatation and filling defect in 4th ventricle; the aqueduct is enlarged. Despite large tumour protruding into the 4th ventricle there was no obstruction of the CSF. passages. The occipital squama had been taken away 7 months previously during exposure and removal of the granuloma, see foregoing Fig. 66 (Case 5. 3)

a tuberculoma with specks of fatty degeneration. The mass was rather poor in blood supply and there were no troublesome "feeders" entering it from the dura or the cerebellum (Fig. 66). The granuloma was eventually scooped out in toto with the finger and without a major bleed, leaving behind a raw surface which was carefully lined with oxycel; a few bleeding points were cauterized. The 4th ventricle was not opened nor was the dura mater on the right side incised. A free flow of cerebrospinal fluid from the patent foramen of MAGENDI was now established. Haemostasis was no problem. The dura was closed easily and completely and the flap re-sutured in the usual way. This surgical intervention was a smooth procedure throughout; the patient had received one pint of blood.

He did very well after the operation and was up and about on the 10th day. The wound healed primarily. On discharge from the hospital, the patient had a resolving papilloedema, a fine nystagmus on lateral gaze, a slight incoordination and unsteadiness of the left arm, and a doubtful ROMBERG's sign with tendency to fall to the left.

The Pathological Laboratory (Dr. VAN DYK) reported that the operative specimen consisted of a torulosis granuloma with giant cells and inclusion bodies.

Seven months later, the man was re-admitted because of persistent vomiting and dimness of vision in the left eye. On examination, he tended to veer left on walking and there was dysdiadochokinesis and hypotonia on the left side. The optic discs were not choked. The lumbar fluid contained 100 mg.-% protein, globulin $++$, whereas sugar and chlorides were within normal limits. A *lumbar air encephalogram* revealed marked dilatation of the ventricular system and a filling defect in the caudal part of the 4th ventricle suggesting a recurrent mass there (Fig. 67). However, since the air had entered freely the ventricles from below, there was no indication of obstruction of the cerebrospinal passages. No operation was advised. The condition, at first, became worse; a paralysis of the 9th and 10th cranial nerves on the left together with a left HORNER's syndrome developed. In addition, there was a suggestion of facial paresis on the left. Under long-term treatment with amphotericin[1] considerable improvement took place, vomiting ceased and all pareses disappeared. Even the cerebellar signs and HORNER's syndrome regressed so much that the patient, after a 10 weeks' stay in hospital, was discharged to be followed up in the outpatients clinic.

Comment. Infestation of the central nervous system with torula histolytica or cryptococcus, on the whole, is not very common. FREEMAN and WEIDMAN (1923) were the first to describe minute multilocular cysts filled with a mucoid substance and giving the grey matter of the brain a sponge-like appearance. From most cases on record so far it is evident that the typical lesion of cryptococcal infection is a wide-spread chronic meningitis or meningo-encephalitis whereas solid, tumour-like granulomas apparent to the naked eye as such and amenable to surgery, are rare occurrences.

Up to 1947 (data derived from G. B. HASSIN, 1947) only five cases of localised torulosis of the central nervous system were described, viz. one in the spinal cord, reported in 1930 by SMITH and CRAWFORD; a cerebellar granuloma; and 3 cases one of which was in the cerebellum and two in the occipital lobe, reported by SWANSON and SMITH in 1944. HASSIN added two cases of his own, one being a vast cerebellar tumour of long standing, eventually merging into an acute stage of high intracranial pressure; in the other patient necropsy revealed dense foci of torulae scattered throughout the brain.

Torulosis of the brain when presenting in a tumour-like fashion appears as a well-defined oblong or roundish mass lying in the subcortical layer and giving the impression as though having arisen from more superficial meningeal lesions. In COURVILLE's Pathology of the Central Nervous System (1950) a fine picture of such granulomas is to be found, occupying, in this case, both frontal poles. A full clinical description of another case involving the left frontal lobe has been given by KRAINER et al. in 1946. Their case, on operative exposure, presented as a mass arising from the meninges and firmly attached to the dura mater simulating perfectly a subfrontal meningioma.

According to FREEMAN, who in 1931 reported on 43 cases of cerebral torulosis, the sites of predilection are the basal and lateral cisterns and the structures around the basal ganglia, the iter, and the cerebellum.

In the case described above an exceptionally large conglomerate and solid torulosis granuloma was found in the left cerebellar compartment; it was about the size of a golf ball and had the characteristic relations to the meninges referred to above, but no attachment to the dura mater. It is worth mentioning that this mass inspite of its size and its site apparently caused clinical symptoms only at a very late stage when the cerebrospinal passages became obstructed and cerebellar coning followed. As it was surfacing and displacing, but not infiltrating, the nervous tissue while practically no intimate relations to the vascular channels were present, an excision in toto was possible and even comparatively easy; however, in view of the preferential spread along the subarachnoid pathways and possible multiplicity of lesions it was little surprise when the patient returned, within a short period, with signs of a recurrent lesion. This is the more remarkable as, at the time of operation, there was no break-through to involve the 4th ventricle or the subdural space.

The case of KRAINER et al. referred to above shows that the differential diagnosis from a meningioma even on exposure may be difficult; in our case, the vertebralis arteriogram was very suggestive of a tumour arising from the tentorium and in the first instance, a meningioma seemed to be quite possible. As in other forms of fungal infection with occasional granuloma formation the differential diagnosis from tuberculosis not infrequently is impossible to the naked eye, and requires histological confirmation.

---

[1] Vide SMITH, G. W.: The treatment of the torula meningoencephalitis with amphotericin. J. Neurosurg. 15, 572 (1958).

Bibliography

ADSON, A. W.: The treatment of cranial osteomyelitis and brain abscess. Ann. Surg. 108, 499 (1938).
— Cerebrospinal rhinorrhoea: surgical repair of craniosinus fistula. Ann. Surg. 114, 697 (1941).
— — and W. McK. CRAIG: The surgical management of brain abscess. Ann. Surg. 101, 7 (1935).
— — and B. E. HEMPSTEAD: Osteomyelitis of frontal bone resulting from extension of suppuration of frontal sinus; surgical treatment. Arch. Otolaryng. (Chicago) 25, 363 (1937).
— — and A. UIHLEIN: Repair of defects in ethmoid and frontal sinuses resulting in cerebrospinal rhinorrhoea. Arch. Surg. 58, 623 (1949).
ALLEN, K. L.: The clinical significance of low cerebrospinal fluid pressure. A thesis presented to the University of the Witwatersrand, Johannesburg. February, 1947.
ANGRIST, A., and N. MITCHELL: Traumatic haemorrhage of the internal capsule. Arch. Surg. 46, 265 (1943).
ASHERSON, N.: Trotter's syndrome and associated lesions. J. Laryngol. 65, 349 (1951).
ATKINSON, E. M.: Abscess of the brain: its pathology, diagnosis and treatment (Hunterian lecture). Lancet 1928, 483.
BALLANTINE, jr., H. T., and C. N. SHEALY: Role of radical surgery in treatment of abscess of brain. Surg., Gynec. & Obst. 109, 370 (1959).
BOTTERELL, E. H., and C. G. DRAKE: Localized encephalitis, brain abscess and subdural empyema. 1945—1950. J. Neurosurg. 9, 348 (1952).
BOYD, W.: A textbook of pathology. An introduction to medicine. 5th ed. Philadelphia: Lea & Febiger 1950.
BROWDER, J.: Craniocerebral wounds. Exteriorization method of treatment. Amer. J. Surg. 62 (n. s.), 3 (1943).
BUCKLEY, P. J., and J. McKINNEY: Hematoma of the brain. New Engl. J. Med. 224, 716 (1941).
BUCY, P. C.: The treatment of brain abscess. Ann. Surg. 108, 961 (1938).
CAIRNS, H.: Injuries of the frontal and ethmoidal sinuses with special reference to cerebrospinal rhinorrhoea and aerocele. J. Laryngol. 52, 589 (1937); Proc. roy. Soc. Med. 35, 809 (1942).
— Penicillin in head and spinal wounds. Brit. J. Surg. 17 (1944).
— C. A. CALVERT, P. DANIEL and G. B. NORTHCROFT: Delayed complications after head wounds, with special reference to intracranial infections., Bristol: John Wright & Sons Ltd. 1947; Brit. J. Surg.War Surgery Suppl. No. 1.Wounds of the head.
— P. DANIEL, R. T. JOHNSON and G. B. NORTHCROFT: Localized hydrocephalus following penetrating wounds of the ventricle. Bristol: John Wright & Sons Ltd. 1947. Brit. J. Surg. War Surgery Suppl. No. 1. Wounds of the head.

CAIRNS, H., and C. DONALD: Diagnosis and treatment of abscess of the brain. Proc. roy. Soc. Med. 27, 114 (1934).
CAUGHEY, J. E., and O. GARROD: Coma and allied disturbances of consciousness in hypopituitarism. Brit. med. J. 2, 554 (1954).
CAWTHORNE, T.: Proc. roy. Soc. Med. 38, 438 (1945).
CHIASSERINI jr., A., and F. CHIAPPETTA: Intracranial abscesses. A diagnostic and therapeutic investigation based on the analysis of 39 cases. Neurochirurgia 2, 152 (1960).
COLLIS, J. L.: The etiology of cerebral abscess as a complication of thoracic disease. J. Thorac. Surg. 13, 445 (1944).
CONNOLLY, C.: Intracranial haematoma concealed by leakage of cerebrospinal fluid. Brit. med. J. 2, 1154 (1956).
CORREA, A., A. P. MORGANTE and M. L. M. TAVARES DE LIMA: Branchiogenic carcinoma with involvement of base of cranium. Rev. paul. Med. 50, 381 (1957). (In Portuguese).
COURVILLE, C. B.: Subdural empyema secondary to purulent frontal sinusitis. A clinicopathologic study of forty-two cases verified at autopsy. Arch. Otolaryng. (Chicago) 39, 211 (1944).
— Pathology of the Central Nervous System. 3rd ed. Mountain View, California: Pacific Press Publishing Association 1950.
— Intracerebral hematoma. Its pathology and pathogenesis. Arch. Neurol. Psychiat. (Chicago) 77, 464 (1957).
— and E. W. AMYES: Late residual lesions of the brain consequent to dural hemorrhage. Report of two cases with old brain stem lesions verified at autopsy. Bull. Los Angeles neurol. Soc. 17, 163 (1952).
— and O. A. BLOMQUIST: Traumatic intracerebral hemorrhage with particular reference to its pathogenesis and its relation to "delayed traumatic apoplexy". Arch. Surg. 41, 1 (1940).
CRAIG, W. McK., and E. M. GATES: Metastatic mycotic abscesses of the brain. Arch. Neurol. Psychiat. 62, 314 (1949).
CRUZ, P. T., and C. F. CLANCY: Nocardiosis, nocardial myelitis and septicemia. Amer. J. Path. 28, 607 (1952).
CUSHING, H.: A study of a series of wounds involving the brain and its enveloping structures. Brit. J. Surg. 5, 558 (1918).
DANDY,W.: Carotid-cavernous aneurysms (Pulsating exophthalmos.) Zbl. Neurochir. 2, 77, 165 (1937).
DIAMOND, I. B.: Brain changes in malignant endocarditis. Arch. Neurol. Psychiat. 27, 1175 (1932).
ECKER, A. D.: Tight dural closure with pedicled graft in wounds of the brain. J. Neurosurg. 2, 384 (1945).
ERASMUS, J. F. P.: Cranial and intracranial pyogenic infections. S. Afr. J. clin. Sci. 1, 301 (1950).

FINCHER, E. F.: Craniotomy and total dissection as a method in the treatment of abscess of the brain. Ann. Surg. **123**, 789 (1946).

FISCHER, E.: Gefäßbedingte Schädigungen bei offenen Hirnverletzungen. Zbl. Neurochir. **6**, 232 (1941).

FOERSTER, O., and W. PENFIELD: The structural basis of traumatic epilepsy and results of radical operation. Brain **53**, 99 (1930); Z. ges. Neurol. Psychiat. **125**, 475 (1930).

FREEMAN, W.: Torula infection of the central nervous system. J. Psychol. Neurol. **43**, 236 (1931).

— and F. D. WEIDMAN: Cystic blastomycosis of the cerebral grey matter caused by Torula histolytica Stoddard and Cutler. Arch. Neurol. Psychiat. **9**, 589 (1923).

GATES, E. M., H. M. ROGERS and J. E. EDWARDS: The syndrome of cerebral abscess and congenital cardiac disease. Proc. Mayo Clin. **22**, 401 (1947).

GRADENIGO, G.: Über die Paralyse des nervus abducens bei Otitis. Arch. Ohrenheilk. **74**, 149 (1907).

GRANT, F. C.: End-results in one hundred consecutive cases of brain abscess. Surg. Gynec. Obstet. **75**, 465 (1942).

GURDJIAN, E. S., and H. R. LISSNER: Deformation of the skull in head injury. A study with the "stresscoat" technique. Surg. Gynec. Obstet. **81**, 679 (1945).

— and J. E. WEBSTER: Surgical management of compound depressed fracture of frontal sinus, cerebrospinal rhinorrhoea and pneumocephalus. Arch. Otolaryng. (Chicago) **39**, 287 (1944).

— — Observations on standardising surgical management of intracranial suppuration. J. Neurosurg. **5**, 1 (1948a).

— — Modern surgical treatment of acute subdural abscess. Arch. Surg. **57**, 411 (1948b).

GUTTMANN, L.: Röntgendiagnostik des Gehirns und Rückenmarks durch Kontrastverfahren. Handbuch der Neurologie, herausg. von O. BUMKE und O. FOERSTER, 7. Bd., 2. Teil, p. 370 et seq. Berlin: Springer 1936.

HASSIN, G. B.: Torulosis of the central nervous system. J. Neuropath. exp. Neurol. **6**, 44 (1947).

HILLER, F.: Die Zirkulationsstörungen des Gehirns und Rückenmarks. Handbuch der Neurologie, herausg. von O. BUMKE und O. FOERSTER, 11. Bd., p. 178 et seq. Berlin: Springer 1936.

INGRAHAM, F. D., and D. D. MATSON: Neurosurgery of infancy and childhood. Springfield, Illinois: Ch. C. Thomas 1954.

IRSIGLER, F. J.: Über den Heilverlauf experimenteller Hirnwunden bei offener und verlegter Knochenlücke. Zbl. Neurochir. **7**, 1 (1942).

— Bemerkungen zum Prinzip und zur Operationstechnik des intrakraniellen Aktes beim Spongioblastom des Sehnerven. Bericht über die Tagung der Vereinigung märkischer Augenärzte am 27. und 28. März 1943 in Berlin. Klin. Mbl. Augenheilk. **110**, 419 (1944).

— Neurosurgical aspects of apoplectic cerebral haemorrhage. (In Afrikaans). Thesis to the Pretoria University. Pretoria 1955.

— Recent experiences with extradural haemorrhage. A paper presented at the South African Medical Congress, Durban, September 1957. S. Afr. med. J. **32**, 187 (1958).

IRSIGLER, F. J.: Intracranial infections of rhinogenous origin. Paper presented at the annual general meeting of National Group of Neurologists, Psychiatrists and Neurosurgeons, Durban, September, 1958. S. Afr. med. J. **33**, 289 (1959).

— Allgemeine Operationslehre. Handbuch der Neurochirurgie herausg. von H. OLIVECRONA und W. TÖNNIS. IV. Bd., 1. Teil. Berlin: Springer 1960.

— and H. SÜDHOF: Untersuchungen über die primäre und sekundäre Infektion experimenteller Hirnwunden. Zbl. Neurochir. **8**, 32 (1943).

JEFFERSON, G.: On the saccular aneurysms of the internal carotid artery in the cavernous sinus. Brit. J. Surg. **26**, 267 (1938).

— Head wounds and infection in two wars. Brit. J. Surg. War Surgery Suppl. No. 1. Wounds of the head. p. 3 et seq. Bristol: John Wright & Sons Ltd. 1947.

— The balance of life and death in cerebral lesions. Surg. Gynec. Obstet. **93**, 444 (1951).

JEWESBURY, E. C. O.: Atypical intracranial haemorrhage with special reference to cerebral haematoma. Brain **70**, 274 (1947).

JOHNSON, R. T., and P. DUTT: On dural laceration over paranasal and petrous air sinuses. Brit. J. Surg. War Surgery Suppl. No. 1 Wounds of the head. Bristol: John Wright & Sons Ltd. 1947.

JOOMA, O. V., J. B. PENNYBACKER and G. K. TUTTON: Brain abscess: aspiration, drainage, or excision? J. Neurol. Neurosurg. Psychiat. **14**, 308 (1951).

KAHN, E. A.: Treatment of encapsulated abscess of brain; visualization by colloidal thorium dioxide. Arch. Neurol. Psychiat. **41**, 158 (1939).

— Brain abscess. In: Correlative Neurosurgery. By E. A. KAHN, R. C. BASSETT, R. C. SCHNEIDER and E. C. CROSBY. Springfield, Illinois: Ch. C. Thomas 1955.

KENNETH EDEN: Mobile neurosurgery in warfare. Experiences in eighth army's campaign in Cyrenaica, Tripolitania, and Tunisia. Brit. J. Surg. **31**, 324 (1944).

KESSLER, L. A., L. G. LUBIC and Y. D. KOSKOFF: Epidural haemorrhage secondary to cavernous hemangioma of the petrous portion of the temporal bone. J. Neurosurg. **14**, 329 (1957).

KING, J. E. J.: Treatment of brain abscess by unroofing and temporary herniation of the abscess cavity with avoidance of the usual drainage method. Surg. Gynec. Obstet. **39**, 554 (1924).

KLAUE, R.: Die indirekten Frakturen der vorderen Schädelgrube beim Schädeldachschuß. Dtsch. Z. Nervenheilk. **161**, 167 (1949).

KOPETZKY, S. J., and R. ARMOUR: The suppuration of the petrous pyramid: pathology, symptomatology and surgical treatment. Ann. Otol. **39**, 996 (1930); **40**, 157 (1931); **40**, 396 (1931); **40**, 922 (1931).

KRAINER, L., J. M. SMALL, A. B. HEWLITT and T. DENESS: A case of systemic torula infection with tumour formation in the meninges. J. Neurol. Neurosurg. Psychiat. **9**, 158 (1946).

KRAYENBÜHL, H.: Cerebral venous thrombosis. The diagnostic value of cerebral angiography. Schweiz. Arch. Neurol. Psychiat. **74**, 261 (1955).

— and Hs. R. RICHTER: Die cerebrale Angiographie. Stuttgart: G. Thieme 1952.

KRAYENBÜHL, H., u. G. WEBER: Zur Behandlung und Diagnose akuter Hirnabscesse und cerebraler Thrombophlebitiden. Acta neurochir. (Wien) 2, 281 (1952).

KRÖNLEIN, R. U.: Vorstellung von drei durch Radikaloperation geheilten Patienten, welche an Hirntumoren litten. Neurolog. Zbl. 29, 107/108 (1910).

KRÜGER, D. W.: Zur Versorgung von Verletzungen im Bereich der vorderen Schädelbasis (unter besonderer Berücksichtigung der Drainage). Zbl. Neurochir. 7, 211 (1942).

— Die offene Hirnabsceßbehandlung nach dem Prinzip der relativen Ruhigstellung des Gehirns. Dtsch. med. Wschr. 75, 542 (1950).

— Die Behandlung der Liquorrhoea nasalis. Acta Neurochir. (Wien) 2, 301 (1952).

— Frontobasale Verletzungen. Mschr. Ohrenheilk. 88, 206 (1954).

— In Beiträge zur Neurochirurgie, herausg. von W. TÖNNIS. Heft 1. Chirurgische Behandlung der frischen Schädelhirnverletzungen. p. 54. Leipzig: J. A. Barth 1959.

KUBIK, C. S.. and R. D. ADAMS: Subdural empyema. Brain 66, 18 (1943).

KUHLENDAHL, H.: Frontobasale Schädelhirnverletzungen und traumatische Liquorfistel. In Beiträge zur Neurochirurgie, herausg. von W. TÖNNIS. Heft 1. Chirurgische Behandlung der frischen Schädelhirnverletzungen. p. 37. Leipzig: J. A. Barth 1959.

LE BEAU, J.: Radical surgery and penicillin in brain abscess. A method of treatment in one stage with special reference to the cure of three thoracogenic cases. J. Neurosurg. 3, 359 (1946).

LEMKE, J. E.: Über Spätabscesse des Gehirns nach Kriegsverletzungen und ihre Behandlung durch Totalextirpation. Zbl. Neurochir. 6, 275 (1941).

— Zur Pathologie und Klinik der Hirnabscesse nach Schädelschußverletzungen. Chirurg 16, 16 (1944).

LINDENBERG, R., and E. FREYTAG: The mechanism of cerebral contusions. A pathologic-anatomic study. Arch. Path. (Chicago) 69, 440 (1960).

LINDGREN, E.: In Handbuch der Neurochirurgie, herausg. von H. OLIVECRONA and W. TÖNNIS, Bd. 2, Röntgenologie. Berlin: Springer 1954.

MEIROWSKY, A. M., and G. R. HARSCH III. The surgical management of cerebritis complicating penetrating wounds of the brain. J. Neurosurg. 10, 373 (1953).

MITCHELL, R. G.: Cerebral venous thrombosis in children and infants. Arch. Dis. Childh. 27, 95 (1952).

NELSON, J.: Involvement of the brain stem in the presence of subdural hematoma. J. Amer. med. Ass. 119, 864 (1942).

NORLÉN, G., and A. S. BARNUM: Surgical treatment of aneurysms of the anterior communicating artery. J. Neurosurg. 6, 634 (1953).

OGILVIE, W. H.: War surgery in Africa. Brit. J. Surg. 31, 313 (1944).

O'CONNELL, J. E. A.: The vascular factor in intracranial pressure and the maintenance of the cerebrospinal fluid circulation. (Hunterian Lecture). Brain 66, 204 (1943).

— Brain fungus. In British Surgical Practice, Vol. 2, p. 344. London: Butterworth & Co. 1948.

ORMEROD, F. C.: Malignant disease of the nasopharynx. J. Laryn. 65, 778 (1951).

PENNYBACKER, J.: Discussion on diagnosis and treatment of cerebral abscess. Proc. roy. Soc. Med. 38, 431 (1945).

— Cerebellar abscess. Treatment by excision with the aid of antibiotics. J. Neurol. Neurosurg. Psychiat. 11 (n. s.), 1 (1948).

PETERS, G.: Spezielle Pathologie der Krankheiten des zentralen und peripheren Nervensystems. Stuttgart: G. Thieme 1951.

PROWSE, C. M.: A case of glomus jugulare tumour with unusual neurological complications. S. Afr. Med. J. 32, 1112 (1958).

RIECHERT, T.: Der „chronische" Prolaps bei Hirnschußverletzungen und seine Behandlung. Zbl. Neurochir. 7, 229 (1942).

RIZZOLI, H. V., W. S. McCUNE and I. J. SHERMAN: Surgical management of metastatic brain abscess. J. Neurosurg. 5, 372 (1948).

ROSENWASSER, H.: Carotid body tumour of the middle ear and mastoid. Arch. Otolaryng. 41, 64 (1945).

ROWBOTHAM, G. F., and A. G. OGILVIE: Chronic intracerebral haematomata: their pathology, diagnosis and treatment. Brit. med. J. 1, 146 (1945).

— and N. WHALLEY: Prolonged compression of the brain resulting from an extradural haemorrhage. J. Neurol. Neurosurg. Psychiat. 15 (n. s.) 64 (1952).

SACHS, E.: A method for exposing the anterior portion of the frontal lobes of the brain. Ann. Surg. 81, 1053 (1925).

— An analysis of brain abscesses observed during the past thirty years. Ann. Surg. 123, 785 (1946).

— Diagnosis and treatment of brain tumours and the care of the neurosurgical patient. 2nd ed. St. Louis: The C. V. Mosby Company 1949.

SCHALTENBRAND, G.: Naturforschung und Medizin in Deutschland 1939—1946. Bd. 81. Neurologie. Teil II (Nervenkrankheiten). Herausg. von G. SCHALTENBRAND. Wiesbaden: Dieterichs'sche Verlagsbuchhandlung.

— Die Nervenkrankheiten. Stuttgart: G. Thieme 1951.

— u. H. WOLFF: Die Erniedrigung des Schädelinnendruckes. Therapie der Gegenwart, Heft 1 (1942).

SCHILLER, F., H. CAIRNS and D. S. RUSSELL: The treatment of purulent pachymeningitis and subdural suppuration with special reference to penicillin. J. Neurol. Neurosurg. Psychiat. 11, 143 (1948).

SCHNEIDER, R. C.: Craniocerebral trauma. In Correlative Neurosurgery by E. A. KAHN, R. C. BASSETT, R. C. SCHNEIDER, E. C. CROSBY. Springfield, Illinois: Charles C. Thomas 1955.

SCHORSTEIN, J.: Compound fronto-orbital fractures (Eight cases.) Brit. J. Surg. 31, 221 (1944).

The Schorstein Lecture on abscess of the brain in association with pulmonary disease. The Lancet, September 18, 1909, p. 843.

SCHREIBER, F.: Cerebellar abscesses of otitic origin in nine children. Eight recoveries after cannulation. Ann. Surg. 114, 330 (1941).

SCHWARZ, H. G., and G. E. ROULHAC: Craniocerebral war wounds. Observations on delayed treatment. Ann. Surg. 121, 129 (1945).

SMALL, J. M., and E. A. TURNER: A surgical experience of 1200 cases of penetrating brain wounds in battle, N. W. Europe, 1944—1945. Brit. J. Surg. War Surgery Suppl. No. 1. Wounds of the head. p. 62. Bristol: John Wright & Sons Ltd., 1947.

— and A. C. WATT: The management of brain wounds in the forward area. Brit. J. Surg. War Surgery Suppl. No. 1. Wounds of the head. p. 75. Bristol: John Wright & Sons Ltd. 1947.

SORGO, W.: Über den primären Wundschluß bei der offenen Hirnverletzung. Zbl. Neurochir. 7, 73 (1942).

SPATZ, H.: Gehirnpathologie im Kriege. Von den Gehirnwunden. Zbl. Neurochir. 6, 162 (1941).

SPERL jr., M. P., COLLIN S. MacCARTY and W. E. WELLMAN: Observations on current therapy of abscess of brain. A.M.A. Arch. Neurol. Psychiat. 81, 439 (1959).

STEWART, O. W., and E. H. BOTTERELL: Cranio-facial-orbital wounds involving paranasal sinuses. Primary definitive surgical treatment. Brit. J. Surg. War Surgery Suppl. No. 1. Wounds of the head. p. 112. Bristol: John Wright & Sons Ltd. 1947.

SYMONS, C. P.: Otitic hydrocephalus. Brain 54, 55 (1931).

— Hydrocephalic and focal cerebral symptoms in relation to thrombophlebitis of the dural sinuses and cerebral veins. Brain 60, 531 (1937).

— Intracranial thrombophlebitis. Ann. roy. Coll. Surg. Engl. 10, 347 (1952).

TAYLOR, H. K.: The Roentgen findings in suppuration of the petrous apex. Ann. Otol. (St. Louis) 40, 367 (1931).

TÖNNIS, W.: Zur Operation der Meningeome der Siebbeinplatte. Zbl. Neurochir. 3, 1 (1938).

— Die operative Behandlung der Siebbeinmeningeome. Chirurg 11, 818 (1939).

— Schußverletzungen des Gehirns. Zbl. Neurochir. 6, 113 (1941).

— Operative Versorgung der Hirnschüsse. Acta chir. scand. 90, 275 (1945).

— Klinische Beobachtungen bei zentralen Störungen der Kreislaufregulation. Dtsch. Z. Nervenheilk. 162, 175 (1950).

TÖNNIS, W., and R. FROWEIN: Liquorfisteln und Pneumatocelen nach Verletzungen der vorderen Schädelbasis. Zbl. Neurochir. 12, 323 (1952).

VARA-LOPEZ, R., and J. SOLIS: Über intrakranielle Luftansammlungen. Ein Fall von Pneumocephalus intraventricularis und aerogenem Abscess. Zbl. Neurochir. 6, 48 (1941).

VILLARET, M., and R. CACHERA: Les embolies cérébrales. Paris: Masson & Cie. 1939.

VINCENT, C.: Sur une methode de traitment des abscès subaigus des hemisphères cérébraux. Large decompression, puis ablation en masse sans drainage. Gaz. méd. Fr. 43, 93 (1936).

VOSS, O.: Die Chirurgie der Schädelbasisfrakturen auf Grund 25jähriger Erfahrungen. Leipzig: J. A. Barth 1936.

WALTHER-BÜEL, H.: Die Psychiatrie der Hirngeschwülste. Acta Neurochirurgica. Suppl. II. Wien: Springer 1951.

WALTNER, J. G.: Anatomic variations of the lateral and sigmoid sinuses. Arch. Otolaryng. 39, 307 (1944).

WATSON, K. C., and G. M. LINES: Brain abscess due to the fungus hermodendron. S. Afr. Med. J. 31, 1081 (1957).

WEBER, G.: Über subdurale Empyeme. Schweiz. med. Wschr. 80, 1349 (1950).

— Der Hirnabscess. Stuttgart: G. Thieme 1957.

WEBSTER, J. E., and E. S. GURDJIAN: The surgical management of intracranial suppuration. Int. Abstr. Surg. 90, 209 (1950).

— R. C. SCHNEIDER and J. E. LOFSTRÖM: Observations on early type of brain abscess following penetrating wounds of the brain. J. Neurosurg. 3, 7 (1946a).

— — — Observations upon the management of orbito-cranial wounds. J. Neurosurg. 3, 329 (1946b).

WERNER, A.: A study of eight surgically treated cases of spontaneous sub-cortical haematoma. J. Neurol. Neurosurg. Psychiat. 17, 57 (1954).

WOLFF, H., and B. SCHMIDT: Das Arteriogramm des pulsierenden Exophthalmus. Zbl. Neurochir. 4, 241 (1939).

WOLMAN, L.: Ischaemic lesions in the brain stem associated with raised supratentorial pressure. Brain 76, 364 (1953).

Subject Index

All numbers signify pages; those in *italics* refer to the figures; numbers printed in **heavy type** refer to the tables.

Tables